The Repetitive Strain Injury Handbook

Robert M. Simon, M.D., and
Ruth Aleskovsky

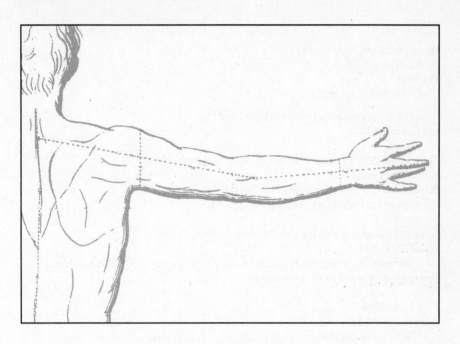

THE REPETITIVE STRAIN
INJURY HANDBOOK
An 8-Step Recovery and Prevention Plan

AN OWL BOOK

HENRY HOLT AND COMPANY   NEW YORK

Henry Holt and Company, LLC
Publishers since 1866
115 West 18th Street
New York, New York 10011

Henry Holt® is a registered trademark of Henry Holt
and Company, LLC.

Published in Canada by Fitzhenry & Whiteside Ltd.,
195 Allstate Parkway, Markham, Ontario L3R 4T8.

Library of Congress Cataloging-in-Publication Data
Simon, Robert M.
    The repetitive strain injury handbook: an 8-step recovery and prevention plan /
Robert M. Simon and Ruth Aleskovsky.
        p.   cm.
    "An Owl book."
    ISBN 0-8050-5930-X (pb)
        1. Overuse injuries Handbooks, manuals, etc.   2. Carpal tunnel
syndrome Handbooks, manuals, etc.   I. Aleskovsky, Ruth.   II. Title.
    RD97.6.S56   2000   99-36203
    617.5'7044—dc21   CIP

Henry Holt books are available for special promotions and premiums.
For details contact: Director, Special Markets.

First Edition 2000

Designed by Kate Nichols

Printed in the United States of America

10   9   8   7   6   5   4   3   2   1

For Isidore Haiblum

who leaps tall buildings at a single bound

Contents

Acknowledgments

This book is the result of countless hours of research and interviews with a great number of experts in various fields who generously donated their time and ideas. With deep gratitude, we wish to thank the following professionals for their contributions (in alphabetical order): A. Benjamin Athon, M.D.; Russell Beasley, L.M.T., senior faculty member of the Swedish Institute School of Massage Therapy; Susanne Chakan, certified hatha yoga instructor; Kira Charles, certified Feldenkrais practitioner; Carleen Clark, R.N.; Edward Clark, M.D.; Sharon Diamond, M.D.; Ruth Dickey, O.T; Robert Fiedler, M.D.; Carolyn Fisher, VESID counselor; Bob Garvey of OSHA; John Kella, Ph.D., ergonomics consultant; Arlette Loesser, O.T.; Susan Nobel, M.S.W.; Pat O'Brien, musician and advisor; Areta Podhorodecki, M.D.; Mark Schmetterer, L.M.T.; Amelia Lee Sheldon, our notable and hard-working editor; Mary Tahan, our invaluable agent; Karen Teeters, P.T.; and Annie Zeybekoglu, illustrator extraordinaire.

In addition to the professionals named above, special thanks go to all the RSI friends who shared their stories, defeats, and successes with us. Our deep appreciation also goes to our many friends who freely gave their advice, humor, support, and, sometimes, computer equipment during the many months it took to finish this book. They helped keep us focused and our spirits high. They are (also in alphabetical order): Paul Aleskovsky, Jean Banks, John dePillis, Kathy Diamond, Ellie Faust-Levy, Kathy Jalbert, Michael Hoffman, Susan Kapit-Husserl, Sam Kaplan, Cheryl Kryzewina, Max and Lila Lerner, Stanley Levine, Jerry Marcus, Jane Margules, Marc Miller, Denise Robert, Renate Schuchardt, Francis Siegel, Phyllis and Arthur Skoy, Elizabeth and Stuart Silver, Judith Ann Yablonky, and George Zarr.

Help must come from all directions when authors create a book of this type. If we have neglected to mention your name, please know that you yourself are not forgotten.

The Repetitive Strain Injury Handbook

PART I

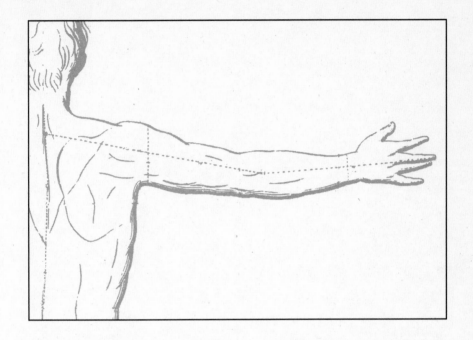

The Eight-Step Recovery Plan

Introduction

Everyone Needs to Understand RSI

Repetitive strain injury (RSI) is a stress-related, cumulative injury resulting from constant repetitive movements. Awkward angles of movement and taking insufficient rest periods are the other culprits that cause this kind of injury. RSI is one of the most misunderstood and misdiagnosed conditions today. With the popularization of technology in our workplace, physicians treating someone with RSI must suddenly consider a whole new panorama of ergonomic concerns. Most doctors know how to *fix* a sprained wrist or broken bone. RSI, on the other hand, is a cumulative condition that can take months or even years to surface with its painful symptoms. The condition, logically, does not respond to any quick-fix approach. An effective treatment plan requires the doctor to identify and help the patient change behaviors that initially produced the injury.

We, humans, are outrun daily by high-speed machines in the workplace. As a result, we push ourselves to our physical limits trying to meet impossible deadlines. With the introduction of the computer, we now type faster than the inventor of the old Remington typewriter ever imagined possible. We communicate endlessly on our cellular phones and through E-mail. We rarely leave our workstations for fear of *falling behind* in the competitive world marketplace. In light of these communication and technological demands, many of us now are constantly *available* and ready to respond. Our bodies are not used to such a nonstop, high-speed schedule. The result is an epidemic of repetitive strain injuries. One in every ten workers filed a workers' compensation claim for RSI during this past year alone. And the numbers are still climbing.

It is time for education. Time to understand our relationship to our jobs and the machines on which we work. Prevention is the only cure for this pernicious kind of injury. It is time to respect our health at work and do the same at home. I hope this handbook will help you and those with whom you work and live to do just that. It is first necessary for you to understand what RSI is and then build your own customized treatment plan to address any RSI symptoms you may now be experiencing.

RSI is a *cumulative injury*—tendons, ligaments, and muscles are worn down over time doing repetitive tasks with few rest breaks. Therefore, the real key to a full recovery goes way beyond being evaluated in a doctor's office and showing up for physical therapy sessions twice a week. Recovery requires a commitment to long-term changes in your attitude and behavior well after you have healed. Hopefully, when you are finished with all eight steps outlined in this book, you will discover new ways to maintain your good health, no matter what you are doing or for whom.

Chapter 1 explains the physiological and psychological changes that can occur when you have repetitive strain injuries. The chapter defines the various kinds of injuries that fall under RSI's rubric and other conditions related to RSI. First, you need a clear picture of what physical changes have occurred and how they impact the rest of your systems (metabolic, cardiovascular, immune, etc.). Then, you can learn how to minimize the symptoms and increase your flexibility, range of movement, and muscle tone. Armed with this new knowledge of RSI, you can ask intelligent questions and create a more effective partnership with your health-care team. The more you understand what is happening to you, the easier it will be to adapt and heal.

Holistic Living Through the RSI Eight-Step Program

This is your guide on how to get the best care, find the most successful alternative therapies to treat your RSI, and adjust to a healthy, productive lifestyle. Ruth Aleskovsky, an RSI survivor, and I, a doctor who has treated hundreds of RSI patients, felt it was important to look at your *whole* life—call it a holistic examination of healthy living—and offer healing suggestions on each and every aspect of your life.

The eight steps we provide here will lead you toward a new and healthier way of living. We hope they will help you take the opportunity to change and continue to enjoy your life during and after your recovery from RSI. We first discuss how you can get a good diagnosis and begin physical therapy and massage. The sooner you recognize your discomfort and pain, the quicker you will recover. After you have found your primary physician for diagnosis and treatment and begun traditional therapy, step three's diaphragmatic breathing techniques will help you to decrease your stress and make all the rest of your recovery easier. Step four, walking off your RSI, brings you further into the proactive format of your recovery plan. This step delves into the whys and wherefores of walking as well as providing an RSI walking plan. Now that you are on your feet and walking, relaxing your muscles with deep breathing techniques that increase your circulation, and releasing muscle spasms, step five provides all the information you need to keep your body fueled and ready to heal. Diet and nutrition can be particularly confusing when you are injured, are low on energy, and have difficulty using your hands and thus have a hard time handling normal routine tasks in the kitchen. Step five gives you concrete suggestions on how to make food preparation easier, teaches you which food choices will do you the most good, and backs up the menu suggestions with solid nutritional basis information. Steps six and seven introduce yoga and exercise routines that will help you get the range of movement you need and not induce pain from your RSI. Included here are warm-ups you can do even at the office or any high-risk situation. Learning your limits in movement, endurance, as well as strength is of paramount importance when you have RSI. To this end a specially designed home limbering and exercise program is outlined for you as well. Suggestions on how to incorporate exercise into your work and daily living routines are described so that these activities become as natural a part of your routine as brushing your teeth.

The last step covers pain management. We tried to define the different kinds of pain you may encounter with RSI and the various treatments available to you. Since most people put off seeing their doctor at the first signs of RSI, the pain cycle is often quite entrenched by the time they begin treatment for this condition. Until this pain cycle is broken, your body can't get the rest it needs to make the most of its natural healing powers. Since everyone is different, having different combinations of RSI and responding at different rates to the pain that results, you will probably have to use a combination of pain treatment therapies during the different stages of your recovery. This chapter gives you the tools you need to get those treatments and decide when it's time to look for new ones.

The eight-step healing program embraces the multidisciplinary approach and is structured so that you can learn and heal at the pace that is best for you. The eight-step plan is designed to optimize your body's natural healing powers and prevent reinjury. Recovery from RSI can be long and arduous. Hopefully, our handbook and eight-step healing program will make your journey back to wellness easier with its attainable, energizing goals.

This handbook is meant to be used in conjunction with your doctor and physical therapist. The information and goals in each of the steps are such that you can work on them at home after you have cleared them with your physician. With your doctor's blessing, these steps should eventually become a way of life for you. Some are easier than others but all will establish healthy habits that will protect you in the future.

Part II of the handbook is told from coauthor Ruth Aleskovsky's perspective. Ruth interviewed hundreds of RSI sufferers all over the country and combined their tips with suggestions and information from leading ergonomic and medical RSI experts to create this section. In Part II, Ruth addresses everything from how to clean your house and tie your shoes, to how to shake hands and even embrace a loved one in a manner that avoids or greatly reduces the possibility of RSI pain. She also includes a special chapter dedicated to the unique concerns shared by women who have RSI. Hormonal fluctuations, osteoporosis, and cancers peculiar to women are often not addressed by doctors unfamiliar with the fact that the life changes women experience greatly impact the various aspects of RSI.

Setting Realistic Goals

Before we make our way through the eight-step healing program, let's stop a moment and think about resolutions, goals, and promises we make to ourselves. This handbook is your guide. These tips should help you personalize each step's techniques and suggestions. Take a deep breath as you read the following tips:

• **Be realistic.** It may be more practical to say you'll do your breathing exercises every other day for the first week than to say you'll do them three times every day. Only make promises you can keep. Make yourself a weekly schedule, then try to stick to it.

• **Be specific.** It is easier to reach a goal when you define it exactly. Instead of saying, "I won't do anything today that will hurt my hands," try defining your goal to "Before I begin a task, I'll think about how to break down the task so I am not working more than ten minutes at a time. I will also stop if I feel any pain or discomfort and I will rest." Everyone is different and has individual needs. I make suggestions in this handbook that you can discuss with your occupational or physical therapist and then adapt to your own situation. One of the simplest but most helpful lessons you can learn in recovering from RSI is often the most difficult to remember: Take the time to discover how you move and what you need to be pain free during each task. And don't forget to take frequent breaks and breathe!

• **Set a timed goal.** If you are trying to break a bad habit, do it one day at a time. If you forget once or twice, don't beat yourself up. Just stop and start again. It takes time and patience to get well.

• **Reward yourself in the process.** Make sure you reward yourself for a job well done. If you make it through a day relatively pain free, fully exercised, or having avoided a bad habit, treat yourself to a special pleasure. You've had years of moving the same way that caused your present injury. The changes are not going to happen overnight. And when they do, you should give yourself a treat. These rewards will help your brain-muscle connection remember what it is supposed to do.

Name the Pain: A Hard and Fast Rule

As we already mentioned, one of the first things you have to do for injuries such as RSI is get an early diagnosis. RSI is cumulative in nature. It can take months or years before you even feel any discomfort at all. It makes sense that an injury that takes so long to become symptomatic isn't going to go away overnight. All the more reason to get that diagnosis as soon as you can and not procrastinate. Many RSI sufferers ignore the discomfort typical of this condition's early symptoms. They hope it will go away. But this is the worst move you could make. If you have recurring pain in your hands or arms and know your days are filled with repetitive motions, make a doctor's appointment immediately. *Name the pain you are feeling.* This is your first step back to good health. Then begin treatment. Don't put off these simple tasks. The pain or discomfort is real and you need to know what is wrong. The pain you are feeling won't go away just because you ignore it. If the pain you are feeling really is the result of RSI, it will become worse and possibly disabling.

The Cumulative Effects of Injury

When you are injured, your whole system is weakened and you can become more susceptible to other diseases and injuries. One of my patients with four different kinds of RSI had great difficulty sleeping through the night regardless of how many pillows or adjustments she made. She responded to her sleep deprivation and stress by overeating. The subsequent weight gain and the constant interruptions in her sleep patterns eventually developed into a condition called sleep apnea. One suffering from sleep apnea falls asleep, stops breathing, and suddenly awakens. The cessation of breathing causes an adrenaline rush that awakens the sleeper with a start. When my patient awakened due to her

sleep apnea, she inadvertently jerked her neck to the side and aggravated the RSI strain in both her neck and shoulder muscles. Again, the
sleep apnea possibly could have been avoided if other symptoms of my
patient's RSI had been addressed as soon as she noticed them.

Don't let this happen to you. Throughout your recovery your symptoms will change constantly. All of them are important. Inform your
doctor of *all* changes you notice. This handbook will give you techniques so you can name your pain and be aware of what is happening as
you start and continue on your treatment plan. If something feels
uncomfortable, find out why.

You must take special care to nurture your entire body when you are
recovering from RSI. The depletion of resources demands that you get
more rest and nutrients of a specific kind. If you don't, your immune system may weaken leaving you vulnerable to other ailments. This book
will tell you how to keep your system nourished with specific nutrients
to help you heal.

Your Handbook Is Your Recovery Tool

In addition to leading you from your first visit to the doctor's office, out-
lining the simple nonintrusive tests physicians use to diagnose possible
RSI, all the way through the healing process, this book also provides you
with the vocabulary and questions that can help as you choose the best
doctors, physical therapists, and alternative therapists for treatment.
Your chosen doctor may suggest you take a few intrusive tests that can
be uncomfortable. In these pages, you'll find tips on how to relax and
reduce the stress of these necessary tests.

Alternative therapies found particularly effective for RSI are also
outlined for you here. These can be as simple as taking a forty-five-
minute walk every day or drinking enough water or warming up your
muscles with a few yoga positions before you sit down to work. They can
involve different kinds of massage and other body-work techniques,
meditation, or new food choices that give you the extra nutrients necessary for soft-tissue healing as well as lifting some of your depression.

Many of the therapies offered here, although they are considered
alternative or *complementary* by many traditional medical practitioners,

have been successfully helping people overcome physical and emotional stress and strain for centuries. Alternative/complementary therapies *round out* your traditional treatments so that, once you recover, you can practice prevention and live with a higher level of energy and less stress.

Why a Multidisciplinary Approach to Treatment?

RSI demands a multidisciplinary approach to treatment for the simple reason that the very cause of the injury is integral to the way you live and work. Repetitive strain injuries are complex in origin. You need to understand the whole picture of your life, your health, and your pain in order to develop a plan that will best insure long-term relief from RSI. Your recovery will entail the actual retraining of muscles and movements that are second nature to you and the very cause of your discomfort. It will demand that you develop a new level of awareness of your work, your body, and your emotions. For that same reason, your doctor can't just treat your wrist or elbow. He must look at the way you live and move. He has to determine *how* you work and play. To do this effectively, he needs a working partnership with you and your therapists. Keep this in mind. You'll want to keep all of the members of your treatment team informed of your condition as it progresses and its treatment for the most effective multipronged approach.

Physical therapy is required but so is learning how to breathe in order for your healing muscles to get the oxygen and nourishment they need. You need to walk to reduce the stress of sitting, decrease your depression, and give your body a chance to maintain its fitness level. You need to break the vicious pain cycle to enable you to sleep deeply on a regular basis and begin to heal. Alternative therapies offer these solutions and more as complements to the traditional physical therapy approach. For those of you without RSI but in a high-risk situation for this condition, this program is a way to stay in optimum health and catch any problems before they turn into disabling pain.

We wrote this handbook to serve as a friendly supportive information guide on your journey back to health. RSI may take a long time to heal. Your recovery will require you to make real changes in your habits and approaches to work and your home. Although this is not always easy, as you integrate each step in your daily life, you should begin to realize that recovery is yours to control. We have included case histories and interviews from real people with RSI, just like you, who were able to overcome their pain, adapt, and heal. One of our main goals is to share information others have found useful in their recovery to save you time and get you out of pain as soon as possible. The habit of rushing and overusing muscles is difficult to break. Patients need the support of their family, friends, coworkers, and employers. I hope these inspirational stories help when the road becomes arduous.

RSI Is Not New

Treating soft-tissue injuries such as RSI is not new. RSI in the form of writer's cramp was diagnosed years ago in monks who worked as society's scribes. What is new is the speed of the machines we use in our work and the use of alternative therapies to address this human-machine interaction. These new therapies address the whole body and the patient's entire scope of activities. In our book, we've researched, interviewed, and compiled experiences to help you heal. Our goal is to make sure that no one else is injured with RSI. For those already injured, it will take work and adjustment, but your symptoms can disappear. You can return to a normal, healthy lifestyle with time and the right care. We hope the ideas and program in this book will hasten your recovery.

Now let's take the first step toward that goal and learn in detail about the different kinds of RSI and how you can recognize its symptoms.

1. What Is Repetitive Strain Injury?

RSI Defined

Repetitive strain injury (RSI), also known as *cumulative trauma disorder*, is an umbrella term that describes over twenty different kinds of soft-tissue injuries. Tennis elbow, carpal tunnel syndrome, tendinitis, and writer's cramp are some of the more familiar types. Many people today suffer from pain in their hands and arms but are unaware of the name or cause of their condition.

Peggy was one patient who, like many others, was confused about the exact nature of her injury. This forty-two-year-old woman lived in a small town north of New York City. She went to three doctors before arriving in my office. After I explained that her diagnosis included a few kinds of repetitive strain injury, she replied that she had no idea what I was talking about. We talked some more. Peggy was familiar with one of her conditions; she had read about carpal tunnel syndrome (CTS) in her local health column but had no real understanding of the other injuries that fell under the RSI umbrella. When they hear RSI, many patients automatically assume they have carpal tunnel syndrome. In fact, CTS makes up only about 1 percent of all repetitive strain injuries.

When Peggy understood that RSI was just the umbrella term—a way for the medical professionals to classify her type of injury—her real education began. It was the beginning of her recovery.

Carpal tunnel syndrome, compression and inflammation of the median nerve in the wrist, is one of the most publicized and most familiar types of RSI as it is often the result of overuse at the computer.

Too many times I hear patients say, "Oh, I don't have RSI, I only have carpal tunnel syndrome. That's not as serious." This is just not true. CTS is one kind of RSI and it needs to be treated immediately.

If you have a chronic pain in your hands and/or arms, it is important to understand exactly what injuries you have and how you were injured. This is the only way you can insure recovery and prevent reinjury especially if you have a cumulative injury like RSI. Express your doubts and fears to your doctor and ask questions. The faster you get answers, the quicker you can begin appropriate treatment. Your doctor needs to know how you feel about your injury and in what ways it affects your daily activities. Each treatment plan for RSI is tailored to each individual patient's needs. You need to participate and offer information to help your doctor create the best plan for you. Expressing pain and discomfort is not complaining. Explaining your symptoms is *your* responsibility in your partnership with your physician and is key to your successful treatment. Speaking up with questions, thoughts, suggestions, and emotions will also help reduce the feelings of vulnerability and helplessness often felt by sufferers of RSI.

Causes of RSI

RSI is the result of long hours spent performing repeated movements with few, if any, rest periods. Its effects can range from slightly painful twinges in the arms and hands to crippling chronic pain. Patients complain of being injured while working at seemingly innocuous activities such as hitting the keys on a computer keyboard or playing the piano. These movements become dangerous when done a thousand times an hour for weeks, months, or years, with few breaks. Leon Fleisher, a renowned concert pianist, was struck with RSI in his right hand over thirty years ago. As a result, he was forced to stop using his right hand. For a long time, Mr. Fleisher had to perform piano compositions written for the left hand only. Today, he is trying to teach prevention to his students so they won't experience the disabling pain from RSI as he did. He says, "I try to tell students to take breaks. There is such pressure to produce perfect sound that practicing for eight hours straight is not at all unusual. We have to find a healthier way to work. RSI changed my career. Prevention is the only cure."

Other Contributing Factors to RSI

In my office, I often see patients who are exhausted, have high-stress jobs, poor posture and nutrition, and usually don't exercise. Sally, a graphic designer, had a day typical of many of my patients. She ran out of her house in the morning with only a cup of coffee for breakfast. She worked a hectic nine-hour day always on deadline. She spent the majority of her day hunched over her computer, her thumb working overtime as she designed using the computer mouse. After work, this thirty-nine-year-old mother rushed home to feed her three kids and help them with homework and then crawled into bed for a mere six hours of sleep—if she was lucky.

Sally's day, perhaps like your own, is filled with the contributing factors to RSI unknown to most workers. A daily routine of stress, food on the run, little sleep, and less than regular exercise can lead straight to RSI. A little awareness can go a long way toward prevention. Small changes in posture, computer-monitor height, and nutrition can be deciding factors between injury and living a healthy, vigorous life. Industry has not yet taken the economic consequences of RSI seriously. But that should not stop you from doing so. Let's take a look at the epidemic proportions to which RSI has risen in the last few years. The need for education is obvious as prevention will save millions in health costs and increase productivity.

RSI Is on the Rise

Workers have been suffering with RSI for a long time but not in the numbers that are appearing today. RSI was first described in 1717 by Bernardino Ramazinni, the father of occupational medicine, as he treated scribes for what we know today as focal dystonia, or writer's cramp. With the advent of technology, the condition of RSI has grown to epidemic proportions among a myriad of professionals including computer users, assembly-line workers, meat processors, cashiers, journalists, and surgeons, to name only a few. The U.S. Bureau of Labor Statistics reports that *8.4 million workers* were stricken with RSI last year alone. Between 1990 and 1997, RSI increased an unbelievable *80 percent*. *The New York Times* has called RSI "the epidemic of the '90s." Experts estimate that the average person faces as much as a *one in ten* chance of eventually developing RSI. Now, approximately 60 percent of workers' compensation claims result from RSI. The average cost per incident of RSI is twelve thousand dollars. And the average workers' compensation claim (with surgery) is over forty-three thousand dollars. Perhaps, as people become more aware of the causes of RSI and education about prevention increases, the rate of occurrence of this condition will decrease.

Everyday Consequences of RSI

The far-reaching everyday consequences of RSI are also hard to fathom unless you know someone who is living with RSI or you have been diagnosed yourself. But once you have experienced it, you realize the importance of prevention.

Below are some typical situations an RSI sufferer may face. These true stories may sound familiar if you have RSI and will help those of you who live or work with someone who suffers from weakness, fatigue, and pain that can cause him to minimize the use of his hands and arms.

• When the pizza finally arrives, a computer programmer takes lunch but lacks the strength to rip the pieces of pie apart.

- A young interpreter for the deaf drops her keys; she didn't feel them leave her numbed hand.
- A two-year-old cries, and his mother can't pick up her child to comfort him as she is unable to support his weight with her spastic, weakened arms.
- A typesetter's husband puts his arms around her shoulders in the movies. She gasps with pain and pulls quickly away.
- At work, a journalist begins to miss deadlines. When his boss asks him to write up a report, he finds his once friendly computer has become an implacable enemy. Now his fingers cramp in pain as he attempts to use the keyboard. For the first time in his life he is unable to do his job properly.

Depression sets in with most RSI sufferers experiencing this kind of pain. One of my patients, Peter, explains, "When I was first injured, I was in a lot of pain. I found myself getting extremely angry and frustrated because no one, including my girlfriend, understood how debilitating it all was. It was as if they kept forgetting about my pain because I looked all right." Peter said his coworkers began to resent him as they were forced to do part of his workload. His feeling of helplessness soon became overwhelming.

Eventually, Peter was compelled to take a medical leave for an extended period of time. His boss was far from understanding, and ultimately, Peter was forced to quit his job. Many with RSI are simply fired. Peter is like many others who find themselves severely injured with RSI—besides feeling lousy, they also become financially vulnerable.

Finally, Peter's luck began to change. After his doctor told him the pain in his hands was from fatigue and all he needed was a vacation, Peter went for a second opinion. This second doctor, who had experience treating RSI, diagnosed him with four different types of soft-tissue injury. Peter was relieved—for the first time he received confirmation that he was injured. With the proper treatment plan, this new doctor told him, the symptoms could be stopped and the injury's effects would be reversed.

As you can see from Peter's case and may know from your own experience, RSI is a condition that not only has to be fought physically but psychologically as well. You have to trust what your body is telling you and address and name the pain, regardless of what others think or say.

Warning Symptoms of RSI

Belief is one of the most important factors when you are recovering from RSI. You need to believe that your pain is real. You need to understand that in order to heal, you must make changes in how you work and live. Acknowledging RSI warning symptoms is your first step toward health. Now let's look at your case.

First, do you suffer from any of the following symptoms?

- Numbness, tingling, or pain in your hands, elbows, arms, or neck
- Lack of motor control or clumsiness in your hands
- A feeling of heaviness or a lack of endurance in your hands or arms
- Interrupted sleep patterns because of discomfort or pain in your hands or arms
- Stiffness or chronically cold hands
- Tenderness to touch (hypersensitivity) in your neck, shoulders, arms, or hands

Now ask yourself the following questions:

- Do you work long hours with few rest periods?
- What are you doing that is different from others doing the same job?
- Has your pain arrived overnight or has it built up over time?
- Do you exercise and eat a healthy diet?
- Is there something you can do right away to lessen the pain and other symptoms?
- Is RSI preventable in your case?
- What can you do to shorten your recovery time?

Think about your answers to all of these questions as you read through the rest of the chapter. This will give you a better understanding of your condition and the treatment of RSI in general.

How Does RSI Start?

The Healthy Body

When you are healthy, your connective tissues (tendons, ligaments, muscles, and nerve sheaths) are similar to ropes in a pulley system. You've been pulling and pushing these ropes for years. They allow you to reach, pull, punch, swing, and type. The lymph fluids and blood lubricate your ropes so they slide smoothly back and forth, making your movements effortless and controlled. Besides keeping your system oiled, these fluids also wash away any unwanted waste. In short, when you move, there is a constant stretch and release happening.

Normally, when a muscle is worked as discussed above, it produces a dozen or so inflammatory metabolics and neurotoxins. These are waste products that are flushed away by the lubricating fluids or blood in your system. Your connective tissues, the ropes in the pulley system, normally break down or tear when you move and then naturally scar and heal when you are at rest. When you limber up before you exercise, these scars are stretched out and the neurotoxin backup is washed away. If you do not, the scarring can shorten your tissues, which results in stiff and tight muscles. If you rest and stretch your muscles regularly, your tendons and ligaments will function smoothly and properly for decades. If not, RSI and other soft-tissue conditions will set in.

The RSI Body

When you overuse your connective tissues, giving them no time to rest and heal, they scar and shorten. Then lactic acid builds up, irritating your tendons and ligaments and causing them to fray. When your connective tissues fray, they also start to swell and become inflamed. As the tendons, ligaments, or sheaths around the nerves swell, they can compress or *pinch* a nerve, which in turn blocks the natural flow of the lactic acid fluids. This waste backup eventually breaks down chemically into a substance that causes the tendons that normally move freely and easily to fuse together. I call this the *gluing effect*. The damaged tissues literally become glued together, sometimes limiting their movement by as much as 50 percent.

One of my patients, Paula, reports how her arms and shoulders feel and I can tell she is experiencing this gluing effect of the tendons. Paula has worked as a grocery-store cashier for over ten years. "All I do all day long is count money and punch the cash register. I couldn't figure out why my arms and hands felt so heavy and tired. I mean, I'm still young [twenty-eight]. All of a sudden, I felt like an old lady!" Paula said to me. She goes on to explain that the pain started slowly with a dull, throbbing ache. Gradually, she began to drop coins and found it impossible to load heavy items into bags while she was packing the groceries. "Everyone was getting mad at me—customers and my boss. So I went to my doctor and he tells me that I have something called RSI."

Paula and I sat together and closely examined her daily routine. Plotting the cumulative effect of her job that culminated in RSI was not difficult. During her ten years, Paula said her days were busy. She had a routine of working long hours, taking short breaks, grabbing a quick lunch, and never doing regular exercises or warm-up stretches. Paula pushed her body beyond its natural limitations. Her overused tissues simply couldn't restore themselves fast enough. Her torn tissues eventually healed and scarred but without the proper stretching and fluid. Thus, they became inelastic and glued together. The scarring shortened her muscles so that it was impossible for her body's pulley system to function normally. This natural tearing and healing happens ordinarily in tissues in every part of your body. But when you have RSI, your body has had no time to rest or nourish itself and therefore your tendons and other soft tissues do not heal. I explained this to Paula and we started working on a treatment plan that included daily stretching and exercise.

Stretching before and after workouts is as important as posture and nutrition. Professional athletes have strict regimens of rest periods for this very reason. During my stint as a professional sports team physician, I emphasized to all the players how important it was to stretch, rest, and eat right. I saw too many athletes get hurt just because they didn't treat their bodies with respect. I also suggested that the athletes rotate their exercise routines giving each area of the body a full day to recuperate. I give my patients who work in an office or at a cash register or on an assembly line the same advice.

Heavy Work—Not the Only Culprit

The overworking of muscles doesn't just happen with heavy-duty work. It can also occur while we are doing something light such as typing, punching a cash register all day, or even playing the violin. Immense amounts of repetition and continual use of the same muscles cause RSI. The muscles don't get enough rest. The lymph fluid doesn't have the chance to clean the system of its waste. People begin to feel discomfort, extreme fatigue, pain, and numbness. But *RSI can take years to build up and may cause no severe symptoms for a long time.* The bright side to this aspect of RSI is that if you catch RSI in its early stages, the damage will be less and your recovery quicker.

CONTRIBUTING FACTORS OF RSI

To assess your risk, compare your habits to the following list of activities or indicators that can contribute to RSI. If you see many items here that coincide with your routine, you might consider changing your habits before pain sets in. Your habits can be the earliest indicators of RSI risk.

- Awkward and/or static postures
- Too much speed, force, and/or duration of movement such as key stroking
- Inactivity such as sitting for long periods slows blood circulation thereby decreasing the efficiency of your muscles
- Lack of frequent breaks
- High-pressure, deadline environment
- Poor nutrition and/or excess weight
- Lack of regular exercise
- Other serious medical conditions such as thyroid disease, arthritis, diabetes, or osteoporosis make you more vulnerable to RSI

The Different Kinds of RSI

Now that you understand the general physiology of RSI, let's look at some of the specifics. Diagnosing RSI can be difficult not only because many other conditions have similar symptoms but also because there are few visible indicators for it. If you've experienced increasing pain in your hands and arms, it is important to find a doctor who takes your pain seriously and who has experience with RSI.

My patient Lynn remembers, "I went from doctor to doctor before anyone diagnosed my RSI. I was beginning to believe that all my symptoms were psychosomatic. One doctor had me almost convinced I was a hysterical woman. Luckily, I persevered and finally found a physician who had experience with RSI and believed I really hurt." Lynn's experience is sadly not an uncommon one. I can't emphasize enough the importance of respecting your feelings. Keep looking until you find the right physician for your diagnosis and treatment.

Dr. Areta Podhorodecki, a physician in New York City who specializes in the treatment of RSI conditions, reiterates the fact that RSI has only recently been recognized by doctors as a legitimate ailment: "A year ago, I would lecture about RSI to an almost empty auditorium. Now there is standing room only. Slowly physicians are becoming more aware and educated as more and more of their patients are complaining of RSI symptoms."

Since it is common for several RSI injuries to occur at once, multiple symptoms may be tricky to pinpoint. Ricky, a taxi driver who usually drove a ten-hour shift, complained of sharp pain that shot down his arms into his fingertips. At first, I was convinced he had carpal tunnel syndrome. However, after extensive testing, I found that he suffered from thoracic outlet syndrome, ulnar nerve compression, and carpal tunnel syndrome. He also had residual arthritis in his neck. Once I properly diagnosed the multiple conditions, I was able to suggest appropriate treatment that addressed all his problems. Each case of RSI must have a careful and complete diagnosis to insure the most effective treatment. You must work with your doctor in order to reach your full diagnosis. Communication is the key.

SOFT-TISSUE PROBLEMS IN A NUTSHELL

Let's look at the soft tissues that are usually injured when you are diagnosed with RSI. As you understand how your body's machine is put together, you can then discover how to talk most effectively to your doctors and therapists about your condition and take steps that will help you heal.

- **Tendons:** Continual irritation causes tendinitis and tendon synovitis.
- **Ligaments:** Chronic tension and irritation can injure ligaments.
- **Muscles:** Overworking muscles causes strain and fatigue.
- **Nerves:** Nerves are protected by sheaths. When these sheaths are inflamed or swollen as a result of overuse, the nerve is said to be pinched or compressed.

Tendons

Tendons connect muscles to bone and have little stretch or rebound. Overuse of tendons causes tiny tears that lead to tendinitis or tendon synovitis. You can have either of these conditions anywhere you have tendons. Tendons are extremely susceptible to repetitive strain injuries. Your shoulders, elbows, and wrists are just some of the common places where tendinitis can occur.

Tendinitis—What Is It?

Tendinitis refers to *inflammation of the tendons that connect a muscle to a bone.* It is the result of awkward or sudden movements over long periods of time. It requires an extended period to heal.

> **CASE STUDY:** Jane was a sign language interpreter in a hospital. After eight months of an exhausting schedule during which she rarely took rest breaks and often worked in cramped static positions at the side of a patient's bed or in other high-stress situations such as the emergency room or labor ward, Jane began to experience achiness, swelling, and shooting pains when she moved her arms. She had a classic case of tendinitis in both wrists and in her left shoulder biceps. Once I diagnosed Jane's condition, I immediately started her

on physical therapy twice a week. However, she really didn't show marked improvement until she took a medical leave of absence from her interpreter position and went on total rest. I also suggested she alternate ice and heat packs on her wrists and forearms several times a day and gentle stretching and rest before and after each activity. Jane's recovery was slow but total since she took her injury seriously and didn't lift anything or gesture with her hands for a few months. She will always be at high risk for reinjury, as all RSI patients are, but now that she is careful to take regular rest breaks, do warm-up exercises, and stretches while she works, we hope to avoid any serious relapse.

Shoulder tendinitis occurs where the biceps muscle inserts into the shoulder joint. A primary symptom of this condition is discomfort when your raise your arm. This particular kind of tendinitis is usually the result of poor posture or repeatedly moving your arm over a surface which is too high or reaching for something that is too far away, such as a computer mouse or a lever on an assembly line.

Rotator cuff tendinitis is associated with overusing the arm while your elbows are pointed away from the body. The rotator cuff is a group of muscles and tendons near the shoulder joint that turns the arm in and out and away from the body. This type of tendinitis can develop as you repeatedly reach for a keyboard that is too high or reach back for a part on an assembly line or down into a pocket.

Three other kinds of tendinitis affect the hand. In the wrist and thumb region, **flexor carpi radialis tendinitis** occurs as you hit the space bar too hard creating tenderness at the base of the thumb. You can also injure the tendons that work with the muscles that are used to straighten the fingers, which is known as **extensor tendinitis**, causing pain near the top of the hand close to the wrist as you hold your hands still in readiness to type or hit the cash register keys. **Flexor tendinitis** causes pain in your fingers as you attempt to bend them. Flexor tendinitis commonly results from excessive finger movement or gripping something like a computer mouse.

Tenosynovitis—Almost but Not Quite Tendinitis

Tenosynovitis refers to *inflammation of a tendon* within *its protective sheath or inflammation of the sheath itself* and feels the same as tendinitis, producing tenderness and pain. When the tendons are overused, they swell. The overuse also causes the lubricating fluid (synovial fluid) to back up and as a result the tendons become painful to the touch and there is sometimes a reddening of the skin. **DeQuervain's disease** is a kind of tenosynovitis that specifically affects the thumb.

> **CASE STUDY:** Jack worked as a draftsman in an architectural firm in Boston. He was constantly reaching for the computer mouse with his thumb to do his work. One day he felt sharp pains in his thumb when he used the mouse or turned a doorknob. He was diagnosed with deQuervain's disease.

Trigger finger (flexor tenosynovitis) is another common kind of tenosynovitis. With trigger-finger tenosynovitis, one of the fingers or digits locks in a bent position as a result of a nodule or ganglion cyst growing on the tendon. The cyst gets caught in the sheath and the finger locks in place.

Ganglion Cysts

The presence of a ganglion cyst can be a precursor to the presence of RSI. It is often a warning sign that your tendon is suffering from too much wear and tear. These cysts are found on the tendon, the tendon sheath, or the synovial lining of the joint. They are often indicated by an ovoid bump, which forms beneath the surface of the skin and is accompanied by weakness and an aching sensation around the raised area. These cysts can appear in four places: on the top of the hand, just above the wrist, on the crease of the third finger knuckle, or on the palm side of the wrist. Ganglion cysts usually don't impair movement or cause much discomfort unless they compress a nerve.

> **CASE STUDY:** Max was a concert violinist who came to my office terrified that his hand was permanently disabled. "My finger just

locked. I couldn't straighten it. It hurt so much when I tried, I actually cried out in pain. That's when I knew I had to do something fast." Although Max was able to return to playing on his concert tours after surgery, he integrated strict warm-up sessions and frequent rest periods to accommodate his new vulnerability to further injury.

Ligaments

Ligaments are *strong fibers that attach bone to bone to form joints*. Some joints are surrounded by a fluid-filled lubricating capsule that allows a range of movement. Overexertion, common among computer users and assembly-line workers, makes people in these professions particularly vulnerable to injury at the elbow and shoulder. Once damaged, the joint becomes unstable and susceptible to recurring injury.

Various tunnel syndromes involve ligaments as well as bones and other tissues. Nerves pass through "tunnels" created by bones, ligaments, and nerve sheaths. Three major nerves are involved in these syndromes as RSI: the median or middle nerve, the radial, and the ulnar nerve. These syndromes differ from tendinitis as they will not heal from rest. The pain from tunnel syndromes tends to be constant and the swelling often occurs at night preventing sleep that is needed for healing.

Carpal Tunnel Syndrome

The carpal tunnel is the bracelet formed by a rigid structure made up of bone and ligament just below the wrist at the heel of the hand. Nine finger tendons, connective tissue, arteries, veins, and the median nerve pass through this tunnel from the arm to the hand. The brain sends impulses through this nerve down the arm to control and direct movement in the thumb, forefinger, middle finger, and half the ring finger. Excessive up-and-down movement causes swelling of the many tendons and the median nerve but the carpal tunnel cannot expand to accommodate the swelling. The median nerve is compressed as a result and the patient feels numbness and tingling and experiences a weakened grip. If you suffer from this condition, you may find yourself constantly dropping things and waking up at night because of the pain. All these are symptoms of carpal tunnel syndrome (CTS).

Pregnancy, thyroid disease, use of oral contraceptives, diabetes, rheumatoid arthritis, and Lyme disease all involve fluid retention and can contribute to carpal tunnel syndrome. It is of paramount importance that your doctor take a complete medical history when making a diagnosis and then treat the primary cause of CTS.

CTS often responds well to aggressive physical therapy and retraining. In advanced cases, surgery may be required to prevent permanent nerve damage. Make sure you have explored all possible alternatives before agreeing to surgery.

Radial Tunnel Syndrome

Radial tunnel syndrome (RTS) occurs with the compression of the radial nerve. The radial nerve, like the ulnar nerve, emerges from the neck area of the spinal nerves or brachial plexus area. The radial nerve runs down the posterior (outside) of the arm into the forearm, hand, thumb, and first two fingers. One of the first signs of this syndrome is pain on both sides of the forearm. Patients with RTS often find it difficult to make a fist, their fingers are weakened, and twisting motions such as turning a doorknob are often painful. Radial tunnel syndrome should be treated immediately as it can cause permanent nerve damage. Depending on how severely the nerve is compressed, doctors may recommend surgery. Physical therapy is suggested as the standard course of treatment.

Muscles—Cramps and Spasms

Overuse of muscles causes strain and fatigue, inflammation and tenderness that makes them prone to spasm. The inflammation of muscles can also compress nerves and irritate the surrounding tissues, including tendons and ligaments. Spasms and cramps are triggered when your muscles go into something called *oxygen debt*. One effective way to relieve the cramp or spasm is to feed your starving muscles the oxygen they need by increasing your circulation and oxygen supply through deep breathing. Walking and gentle stretches also help provide your extremities with oxygenated blood. Although you may have a cramp or spasm in your hand, the most effective treatment involves your whole body. Deep breathing, walking, and gentle stretches address your whole system and get it moving thereby releasing your general tension, nurturing all your tissues with oxygen, and releasing any backed-up lactic acid.

> **CASE STUDY:** Lynn came to my office complaining of sudden cramping in her neck and hands. The pain was so acute it made her gasp. "I'd be in the middle of a conversation with my boyfriend and suddenly my hand cramps. It actually curls up. I can't seem to stop the pain and can't straighten my hand. It is like having a painful runner's cramp except in my hand." After a few yoga lessons that I suggested she take for her painful condition, Lynn had learned deep-breathing techniques and was able to release her muscle cramps and spasms when they occurred. She began physical therapy, which taught her stretches and warm-up exercises that increased circulation and kept her relaxed while she worked. She also rearranged her workstations and took more frequent breaks during the day to give her hands a chance to rest and relax.

Circulation, Muscle Strain, and RSI

Poor circulation caused by spending too much time in one position, as well as poor posture, also contributes to muscle strain. During strenuous exercise or overuse during work, your muscles quickly deplete the supply of oxygen that breathing and blood circulation supply. If oxygen is not present in your muscles, glucose is converted to an intermediate molecule called lactic acid, which causes muscle fatigue. In this state of fatigue, muscle fibers cannot contract efficiently and any contraction that does occur may become painful. After ordinary strenuous exercise, the respiratory rate and heart rate remain high for a time. They only gradually return to normal after the body converts the lactic acid back to glucose.

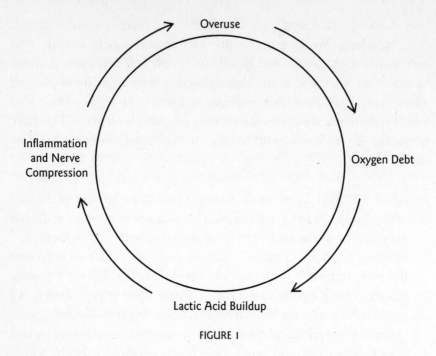

FIGURE I

The muscles in those suffering from RSI never have a chance to convert the lactic acid to glucose and the body remains in oxygen debt. Figure 1 illustrates this cycle. Diaphragmatic breathing techniques (see chapter 4) are beneficial because they provide the RSI sufferer the intensive influx of oxygen the body needs to relax and rejuvenate.

Nerve Compression in Your Neck, Spine, and Shoulders

Many doctors believe that 85 percent of repetitive strain injuries originate from the neck region. It really comes as no surprise since the nerve pathways travel from our upper spine to our fingers and problems anywhere along these long pathways can trigger RSI-related symptoms. Nerve irritation or muscle spasms around the nerves in the neck, for example, can cause numbness or pain in the hands and wrists.

Thoracic Outlet Syndrome

We know that for your muscles to remain healthy they need a constant supply of oxygen-rich blood. The thoracic outlet is a triangular area found above the shoulder between the collarbone and neck. Blood vessels and nerves support the blood flow through this area. When both arteries and nerves are compressed, the result is thoracic outlet syndrome. Symptoms include tingling and numbness down the arm and difficulty holding the arm up as you might do while driving a vehicle or holding a hair dryer.

Ulnar Nerve Syndromes

Sulcus ulnaris syndrome is simply a condition affecting the inside of the elbow near the bone. People who constantly lean on their elbows are likely to develop this syndrome. As the ulnar nerve is compressed it cuts off the blood flow causing a loss of sensation, numbness, tingling, muscle atrophy, and sometimes the ring and pinkie fingers will bend like a claw. Sulcus ulnaris responds well to aggressive physical therapy. Only in advanced cases is surgery advised.

Cubital tunnel syndrome attacks people who work with their elbows bent at right angles for long periods of time entrapping the ulnar nerve in its pathway in the underarm. Symptoms include loss of sensation, numbness, tingling, and muscle atrophy. This syndrome can be caused by epicondylitis, or tennis elbow, where the arms are also held too high for too long, inflaming and swelling either the inside or outside part of the elbow. When one area is weakened by injury, other muscles and tissues take over making us vulnerable to other kinds of injury. The whole nerve pathway can easily become aggravated, causing different kinds of RSI.

Guyon's canal syndrome, also called ulnar tunnel syndrome, is the compression of the ulnar nerve in the wrist near the carpal tunnel. Symptoms include numbness in the ring and little fingers, difficulty grasping objects, and an inability to bend the wrist up and down. A double crush occurs when there is more than one tunnel syndrome around the same area, such as carpal tunnel and Guyon's canal.

Cervical Radiculopathy—Telephone Syndrome

This condition occurs most often in people who hold the phone to their ear with their shoulder as they work. Sales people, chefs, computer users, and mothers—really anyone who is trying to talk on the phone while involved with another task—are vulnerable to this painful syndrome. Holding your head at this awkward angle compresses the cervical discs in your neck and leads to weakness in the shoulder and upper arm as well as numbness in the fingers. Poor posture also contributes to this syndrome.

Double-Crush Syndrome

The double-crush syndrome occurs when a nerve is compressed in two places, often in the neck or thoracic outlet and then farther down in the hand or wrist. Staring at a computer monitor while typing for hours or at a film editor's screen while manipulating a computer mouse can easily bring on a double-crush syndrome. Both activities keep the head and neck in one position for hours while the arms are held steady and the fingers barely move in micromovements. Breathing can become shallow creating oxygen debt, which adds to the stress and tension in the muscles. Then the sheaths around the nerves can swell and entrap the all-important nerves. This syndrome can aggravate the entire nervous system of the upper torso producing severe pain and numbness.

Tension Neck Syndrome

This is marked by stiffness, muscle spasm, and radiating pain. It may start with burning on the back of the neck and trapezius muscles and escalate into sharp shooting pain down into the wrist and fingers. It is caused by any activity where your neck muscles don't move for long hours at a time such as driving long distances without a break, working at a computer screen, or sleeping in awkward positions. Other contributing factors can be lack of exercise and poor posture involving a stance where the head is not aligned with the spine such as bending over a conveyor belt on an assembly line or decorating pastries in a bakery.

Epicondylitis—Tennis or Golfer's Elbow

There are two kinds of common elbow problems that can result in RSI: one affects the outside of the elbow or lateral side, and the other affects the inside or medial part of the elbow. If the pain is on the inside, you might hear it called tennis, pitcher's, or bowler's elbow as the injury is often suffered among those who play those sports. Epicondylitis of the medial elbow occurs when the elbow is raised too high and for too long. But it doesn't just plague sports enthusiasts. If you work in an office or a kitchen, you might want to double-check the height of your desk or work counter. Make sure you aren't holding your arms too high when you work. Play with the heights in your work space by adjusting your chairs or the actual height of the counter itself. Stand on a stool and see if you feel a relief—perhaps from a strain of which you were unaware.

The other kind of epicondylitis, that affecting the outside of the elbow, results from the same form of awkward movement. Patients experience extreme pain when attempting to straighten their arms or contracting them against resistance. The area around the elbow is tender to the touch. Graphic designers and other heavy mouse users seem to be especially at high risk for this condition.

Raynaud's Disease

Raynaud's disease is marked by blood-vessel constriction in the fingers, which often renders them cold, pale, and painful. This phenomenon is five times more common in women than men and usually affects both hands and can be accompanied by tingling and numbness. Anything that promotes further constriction of the arteries such as smoking or the use of drugs such as beta blockers, clonidine, and ergotamines can aggravate Raynaud's disease and should be avoided by those who suffer from this condition.

Focal Dystonia or Writer's Cramp

This is the involuntary cramping of the hand that occurs as a result of misfired signals from the brain. The condition will grow progressively worse without treatment and can be quite frightening to those who have it. Your doctor may ask if you are having trouble with your handwriting or find yourself making involuntary movements with your fingers. This is a serious condition that often plagues instrumentalists (violinists and pianists). Like most RSI, it benefits from early detection and treatment.

Associated Disorders

Here are a few other disorders you and your doctor should be watching for if you have been diagnosed with RSI. They often are mistaken for, accompany, result from, or aggravate RSI.

Bursitis and osteoarthritis: Some joints are cushioned by bursae, fluid-filled sacs that help pad unprotected joints and unsheathed tendons from bone. Bursae permit the tendons to slide easily as the bones are moved. If a joint is used excessively, the bursae may become inflamed and painful. This condition is called *bursitis*. Bursitis commonly occurs near the shoulder joint and can cause pain and impaired movement.

Osteoarthritis, a degenerative joint disease, is one of the oldest and most common types of arthritis. It is characterized by the breaking down of cartilage, which causes the bones to rub against each other. If severe, it can cause loss of movement. The Arthritis Foundation estimates that 20.7 million Americans, over age forty-five, suffer from osteoarthritis. This condition, like Raynaud's disease, affects more women than men. Inflammation, morning stiffness, pain increasing with exercise, and diminished range of movement along with cracking or grating sensations are clear signs of osteoarthritis. Exercise is the best way to prevent any kind of arthritis from worsening. Specifically, warm-water aerobic exercise is one of the most effective ways to keep both bursitis and osteoarthritis safely at bay without aggravating their uncomfortable symptoms. Weight control to prevent extra stress on weight-bearing joints is also recommended.

Whether or not osteoarthritis and bursitis can be classified as RSI is under debate. However, they often accompany RSI or are mistaken for other forms of RSI.

Fibromyalgia: Though not a form of RSI, fibromyalgia has similar symptoms to those of repetitive strain injury. Its trademark is eleven or more *trigger points*, namely painful sites on the body that are tender to the touch. Symptoms include pain that can increase with improper exercise, morning stiffness, fatigue, and diminished range of motion. Cold, humidity, and stress seem to worsen the symptoms. Warm-water exercise, yoga, and walking seem to help alleviate some of the symptoms. Nonsteroidal anti-inflammatories and other painkillers have proved to be ineffective.

Reflex sympathetic dystrophy (RSD): RSD is a complex pain syndrome resulting from trauma, like RSI. It is also triggered by injuries that are followed by a period of immobility as is the case with many RSI sufferers. RSD develops slowly in my RSI patients. Burning pain, an exaggerated response to painful stimuli, experiencing pain triggered by stimuli not usually associated with pain such as touch, tremors, spasms, weakness, and involuntary movements in your arms or hands are common with this condition. A bone scan can also prove the existence of RSD. Traditionally, physicians require the presence of five or more of the above symptoms before diagnosing RSD in a patient. However, recent literature shows the benefit of treatment when RSI patients experience only three of the above symptoms, labeling the condition "mild" or "early" RSD. Symptoms such as burning pain, which typically takes months for recovery with physical therapy and conservative pain management, have disappeared in a matter of weeks with earlier intervention of aggressive physical therapy and pharmaceutical pain management such as Neurontin, Tegretol, alpha and beta blockers, clonidine, antidepressants, and anti-inflammatories in different doses with varying combinations of each.

Unless RSD is diagnosed and treated within six months of onset, it is likely to worsen and become chronic. A pain-management physician with RSI/RSD experience can make the best pharmaceutical decisions for you. It is also imperative that anyone with RSD increase his level of movement as immobility causes the disorder to progress to a more advanced stage. It is, admittedly, a delicate task to balance the level of movement so as not to cause RSI flare-ups and still move enough to retard the progress of RSD. If you are diagnosed with RSI/RSD, your physical therapist can help you to create a healthy relationship between the needs of these two conditions. Myofascial release, acupuncture, yoga, and extra massage therapy have also proved to be especially effective for those with RSI/RSD.

A note for polio survivors: A recent report published by a Canadian scientist, Dr. Alan J. McComas, a neurologist at McMaster University in Hamilton, Ontario, found that polio survivors lost motor neurons in the spine at a higher rate because of early damage caused by the polio virus. To compensate for this loss, the remaining healthy neurons send out sprouts to reconnect the muscle fibers orphaned when their motor neurons were killed. These neurons may have been carrying *five hundred times their normal workload*, causing the muscle weakness and pain. Polio survivors are 85 percent more likely to have some kind of overuse syndrome than those who never contracted polio.

What this means in terms of exercise, work, and general movement is that the post-polio muscles are working at least twice as hard as those not affected to compensate for the dead or atrophied muscles creating the perfect environment for RSI. This is coupled with the fact that research shows most polio survivors are overachievers. In order to overcome the original polio virus, the patients were taught to fight through pain. Carried through life, these behaviors put polio survivors at extremely high risk for RSI. When a polio survivor exercises, the minute there is a "burn" from exercise or fatigue or pain, he must simply stop. This will enable him to exercise in a healthy, safe way. Dr. Nancy Frick, a leading expert in post-polio syndrome, advises that "for those who do slow down, the pain will subside."

Don't Diagnose Yourself

Now that you have educated yourself about all the common symptoms and types of RSI, relax! Don't diagnose yourself. The information we have shared in this chapter will give you a vocabulary with which to discuss your diagnosis and treatment plan with your doctor. Use this knowledge as a tool to help yourself back to health. Let's review an outline of your course of action. Do any of the symptoms we've discussed apply to the sensations you've had in your hands and arms? If so, follow up with the process of naming your pain and obtaining a diagnosis immediately.

Treatment of RSI and What to Do Immediately

- Get a diagnosis and start treatment as soon as you sense something is wrong. Not knowing is worse than knowing.
- Understand that there are many different kinds of repetitive strain injuries and they often trigger one another.
- Know that when caught early, much of the RSI damage can be reversed.
- Try to discern where your overuse occurs so you can modify your movements and work area. This is the only way you will be able to prevent reinjury.
- Be aware that RSI accumulates over months and perhaps years before symptoms appear.
- Believe you will get better!

2. Step One: Get an Early Diagnosis

As we've mentioned earlier, the keys to a successful and quick recovery from RSI are an early diagnosis and immediate treatment. Without early intervention, people with RSI will continually reinjure themselves. If left untreated, a relatively benign injury can turn into a permanent disability.

The goals of this chapter are deceptively simple:

- Get a complete diagnosis
- Schedule the appropriate tests
- Start a medical journal

Most of my patients have had great difficulty admitting something is wrong and actually making that first, all-important appointment with a doctor.

Alex is a typical RSI sufferer. Let's take a look at why he didn't get an early diagnosis, what the consequences were, and how you can avoid similar pitfalls.

Alex is a thirty-eight-year-old truck driver whose whole business is based on meeting deadlines. He works six days a week driving a twenty-two-foot truck at top speed as he moves loads from one coast of the country to the other. He stops only to grab some greasy, heavy starchy food at various roadside truck stops. On his day off, Alex plays baseball with his sons and enjoys his hobby, woodworking, for which he uses heavy, vibrating tools. What Alex does not know is that even while practicing his hobby, as he uses the various electric tools he is subjecting his hands to vibrations similar to those of the steering wheel he holds all week. In addition, the position of his shoulders, arms, and hands during all of his leisure activities are too similar to his daily work movements to afford his tired body any rest.

Given Alex's habits, RSI was almost inevitable. And he did develop it, but Alex felt symptoms of RSI for over a year before he saw a doctor. He explains, "I just didn't have any time before then. Now the pain's so bad I can barely lift my kid or swing a bat. And driving my truck is out of the question. I can't even ride without pain while my wife is driving. I don't know how it got so bad so quick."

In reality, Alex started feeling sharp pain back in February. However, it wasn't until December that he admitted something might be wrong and saw a doctor. For almost a full year, he would complain to his wife of fatigue, numbness, and sharp pain in his hands and talk about how he found it increasingly difficult to turn the big wheel of his truck while driving. Every time Alex got behind the wheel, used a saw, swung a bat, he unknowingly compounded his injuries. All these activities caused strong vibrations and forced him to hold his arm up high.

After so many years of overuse, Alex's system finally began to weaken and break down. Like most of my patients, he tried to rationalize the pain away. As is commonly the case, Alex found it emotionally easier to deny the pain than to recognize what he was feeling and do something about it. As a result, only after two years of treatment did most of his symptoms disappear. Now, Alex still has to be careful and occasionally has bouts of weakness and recurring tendinitis. If he had consulted a physician earlier, he most likely would have recovered in a few months and had little residual pain.

Denial

One of the major reasons most people like Alex don't get an early diagnosis is *denial*. The period of denial is one of the most dangerous stages of RSI and almost everyone who has this condition goes through it. The shorter your denial period, the better. RSI is a difficult injury to recognize since there are no visible signs of the damage tendons, nerves, and muscle undergo because of it. It just hurts and most of us are all too willing to disregard pain until it becomes unbearable. To hasten your quick and complete recovery, acknowledge any pain you feel in your hands and arms. If you suspect you may have RSI, seek treatment immediately. Don't make the same mistake of procrastination Alex and so many others do.

In order to get past your denial and into treatment, it helps if you understand what is causing your fear. Denial creates a vicious cycle that leads to more pain, more procrastination, and more rationalization as you try to convince yourself there is really nothing wrong. The building pain and fatigue quickly lead to depression and inactivity. For many, the repetitive motions that cause RSI are such a big part of their job and life that they can't even begin to think how they would adjust if they could no longer type, drive, work on an assembly line, sign, or play an instrument. You may have been trying to avoid this very train of thought, afraid of how it will affect your ability to earn a living or do what you most enjoy. But the longer you deny your pain, the more damage you do to your body and the longer it will take to diminish your symptoms and bring you back to a healthy state. When you break through denial, you have a real chance at a full recovery.

Below are the escalating phases denial may drag you through when you have the beginning symptoms of RSI. Read this carefully and try to remember exactly when you went through each phase and what made you move to the next. If you've just started feeling discomfort and haven't been drawn into full denial, get to a doctor before the process starts! The more you understand yourself, no matter where you are, the easier recovery will be. A doctor's clear explanation of your diagnosis, prognosis, and treatment options will be the empowering tools that will help you end denial's vicious cycle, and your denial and fear will be replaced by facts and concrete treatment.

Phases of Denial

1. You began with months or years of overuse of your arms and hands. The damage is cumulative and your symptoms are dormant.
2. Your symptoms begin to emerge slowly but are still easy to ignore. You rationalize that what you feel are everyday aches and pains. Nothing to worry about. Nothing to act upon.
3. Then discomfort and pain become more constant. The damage continues. The discomfort is harder to ignore.
4. Fear grabs hold. You suspect something is really wrong. You really hurt. Weakness, shooting or throbbing pain, burning sensations, and difficulty of movement begin to interfere with your daily routine. You can't do the things you want to do.
5. Should you fight or flee? Flight instinct takes over. Your fear wins and you flee. You try to ignore the pain.
6. Your pain continues to worsen and you awake three or four times during the night.
7. Fatigue and depression set in. You feel overwhelmed. But you still do not act.
8. You try to adjust and compensate for your sudden limitations. Your other muscles begin to tire as you favor the hurting arm or hand.
9. The old adage, "No pain, no gain," kicks in. You decide you can beat this on your own. More exercise. Work harder. You are angry—how dare your body betray you like this!
10. Nothing seems to help. You are scared, cranky, tired, and in constant pain. You get to a point where you just wish this would all go away. You become more and more inactive. Apathy sets in.
11. Pain increases to the point where you can't function. You are embarrassed and desperate. You reluctantly decide to seek medical help.

12. At the doctor's office, denial and reality confront each other. You receive the diagnosis of RSI.

13. You hear what your physician says but don't fully accept the meaning. You believe there really is a "quick fix." You indulge in partial denial for a few weeks or months, continuing habits that reinjure and worsen your condition.

14. Finally, you begin to understand the extent of the damage and admit you are seriously injured.

15. You begin to educate yourself and decide to take an active role in your recovery. You time each activity during your day and take frequent rest periods.

16. Denial is no longer an option. You adopt healthier habits at home and at work. You eat a more nutritious diet, exercise regularly, and find time to relax.

Be Proactive

Wouldn't it be easier if we could just skip from the first sign of pain to diagnosis and treatment? That's what being proactive means. Act now. Worry later. The amount of RSI damage would dramatically decrease and the chance of a speedy recovery increase if you did just that. However, denial is difficult to overcome because it is so strongly intertwined with self-image. Many people think that they are immune to a disabling injury or illness such as RSI. They truly feel that if they ignore the pain, it will disappear.

When the first signs of RSI appear, it is much easier to ignore than to recognize. We all get tired. Minor aches and pains are not all that unusual and go away with a good night's rest. It is when the discomfort and pain doesn't go away that you have to stop and push through your fear. When a pain in your hands or arms continues beyond a few weeks you simply need to find out what's wrong.

The only way to get past the denial stage of RSI is to ignore the arguments going on in your mind. Many patients come into my office with the same kind of story. "I felt like I was going crazy. The pain kept moving. Some days my neck hurt, some days it was my arms and hands. It moved so much that I was sure it would go away if I was just patient. But when it hurt, it really hurt. I honestly didn't know whether or not to go see a doctor. Yes, no. Yes, no. It was like a walking nightmare." If this sounds familiar, wonder no more. Go to the doctor. And, go ahead, complain. Give yourself permission. *It's appropriate.* The pain is *real.* Your body is telling you it needs help. Give it what it needs.

If you hear from your doctor that the diagnosis is RSI and you managed to catch it in the early stages, you should feel relieved and terribly proud of yourself. You will recover quickly. You are taking care of yourself brilliantly. Congratulations! If your RSI is more advanced, according to your doctor, take this time to commit to a recovery plan immediately. Then be proud that you have taken your first step toward recovery.

Common Symptoms of RSI

Here are some questions to ask yourself if you've been feeling pain you suspect is RSI. If you answer yes to four or more, go see a doctor at once. The best way to break through your feelings of malaise and helplessness about any pain you have is to *do something to help yourself. Be proactive.* A simple doctor's visit will start to answer all your worrying questions and, if necessary, put you on a path to recovery. It is truly better to know than to live in ignorance. Getting diagnosed is your first and, perhaps, your most important step.

1. Do your arms feel heavy at any time during the day?
2. Do you have any tingling, feelings of numbness, or pain in your neck, shoulders, arms, or hands?
3. Are you having trouble sleeping through the night?
4. Are packages and books suddenly feeling too heavy?
5. Are you dropping or spilling things more than usual?
6. Do you feel clumsy or awkward?
7. Is it suddenly more difficult to write?
8. Are you having difficulty lifting your arm or reaching behind you?
9. Do you find yourself holding your wrist or rubbing your arm, hand, or neck more than usual?

Start a Symptom Journal

Because pain associated with RSI often travels or changes from throbbing to burning to sharp pain, it is hard to describe where it strikes and what it feels like when you are at the doctor's office. Given this fact, an easy way to help get an accurate diagnosis is to start a symptom journal. Most people with RSI groan at the thought of doing any more writing. However, this can be done with minimal amount of stress or discomfort. I usually recommend that my patients get a lightweight date book that has plenty of room for notes. Using the method of *headlining*, you can jot down the kind of pain (sharp, dull, throbbing, burning, shooting), the location on the body, when it occurred (home, work, transportation), and the situation (typing, driving, cooking, sleeping) near the designated time slots. Use short words and lots of abbreviations. I also ask

---

SYMPTOM JOURNAL SAMPLE

Below is a day's sample entry in a symptom journal.

Monday, Jan. 23
[key: pn=pain; shrp=sharp; shtng=shooting]
8 A.M.: cook brkfst; shrp, shting pn; tired
9:30: bus: yes, pn
10:00: work: type, unbearable pn; had to stop; filing; drop paper; felt clumsy
12:00: lunch: too tired to eat
1 P.M.: type—ouch
3:00: rest; tingling, burning neck and arms; arms heavy
5:00: home: arms tired; drop package
5:30: pick up kids; hdache; neck hurt shrp pn
6:00: laundry can't
7:00: dinner takeout; wrist hurt with fork; hands weak
8:00: pencil: write; handwrtng messy; hurt
10:30: sleep; wke 3X; tingling numb rt arm; cry

Each day, it's important just to highlight the activities that are most uncomfortable. Set up a method of shorthand that you understand and are most comfortable with. A journal will also help keep your progress in perspective.

---

that patients note whether or not they are sleeping through the night. This journal helps with the changing needs of the treatment plan as well as with the initial diagnosis.

Another Way to Track Your Pain

On the following pages you will find three figures. Two represent your front and back. I recommend that you go to a copy shop and make four months' worth of the figures, which means sixteen copies. At the end of each week, sit down with your figures and map out your pain. I've filled in one figure as an example. (See figure 2.) Keeping track of your pain will serve two purposes. It will help you identify where you hurt and what kind of discomfort you are experiencing. And, as you progress through treatment, it will also illustrate when and how you are healing. Recovery can be extremely subtle and difficult to spot if you are not doing something like this that will help you identify it.

In this way, you and your doctor can track your pain and discomfort and pinpoint what activities most aggravate your condition. Your physician and occupational therapist will also be interested in these figure maps as they will help them devise better treatment plans and help with your daily living skills.

The Diagnosis

You, like many people, may hate the uncertainty of a doctor's visit. One of my RSI patients, Donna, admitted, "I hate going to the doctor for anything. It's like opening a Pandora's box for me. I figure once a doctor starts looking around, he's going to find a whole bunch of things that would be just fine if left alone. Somewhere along the line, I did start to think to myself that the treatment is worse than the pain. But it was so severe that I couldn't move. I had to do something. But was I scared! Then my husband and I researched my symptoms on the Internet. The more I learned, even though I wasn't sure of the diagnosis, the less scared I became. I also found out what would happen when I went in for a diagnosis—the nurse was really nice on the phone. So, I figured it was

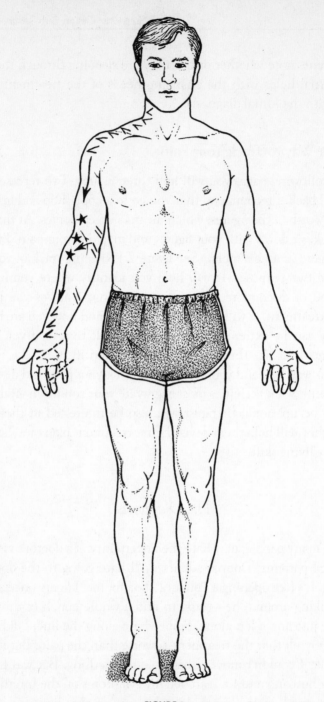

FIGURE 2

** = dull, throbbing pain   // = tingling   ——— = numbness   >> = sharp, shooting pain

This patient has dull, throbbing pain in his arms (***), tingling around the ulnar nerve on the outside of his right forearm (//), numbness in his right hand, ring finger, and pinky, (----) and sharp, shooting pain that starts in his neck and travels to his fingers(>>).

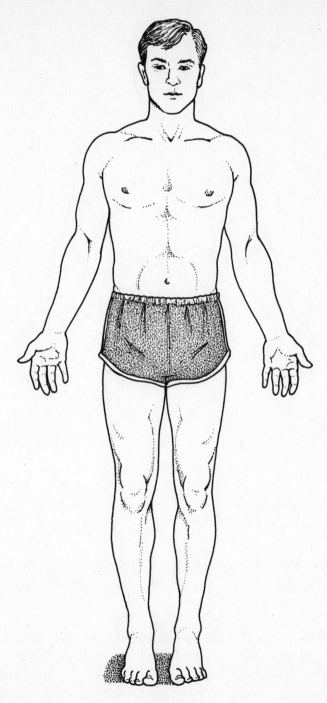

FIGURE 3

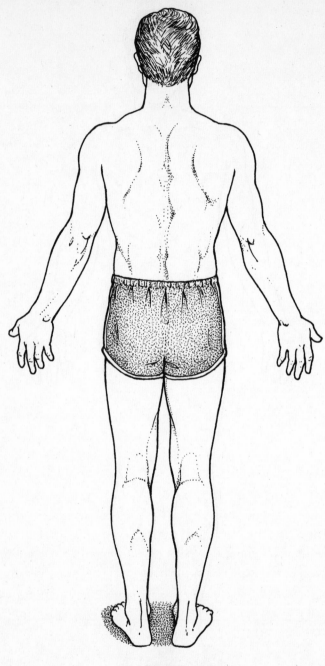

FIGURE 4

better to know what was going on instead of living with this unbeliev-able pain. I'm glad I did. The fear was much worse than what actually happened."

You, like Donna, will most likely feel reassured and a bit more at ease once you know what to expect at your first doctor's visit for what might be RSI. What questions will the doctor ask? What tests will he perform or schedule?

Here's What You Can Expect in the Doctor's Office

• **The questionnaire:** You will be asked to fill out an initial ques-tionnaire that includes a brief medical history if this is your first visit to this doctor's office. Don't be afraid to ask the receptionist or nurse to help you write if you are in pain. That is one of his or her responsibili-ties. You might mention that you will need help when you make the appointment so they will be prepared to assist you when you arrive.

• **Insurance:** Bring all your insurance cards and information to the doctor's office with you. The receptionist will photocopy your cards and return them to you.

• **The initial exam:** The doctor or nurse usually takes your blood pressure and weighs you. These factors are base readings that signify basic overall health and are thus important to monitor during your recovery period. Both may fluctuate because of stress involved with RSI. You need to know what levels are normal for you. This information will help you as you begin to retrain your muscles and adapt to a healthier lifestyle.

• **Nonintrusive tests for RSI:** These tests don't involve any needles or sharp pain. The trick here is to relax and tell the doctor if there is any pain or discomfort when you move. And remember to breathe. Many patients tend to hold their breath when they are tested. Breathing helps you move easier and with less stress. Share information from your symp-tom journal if you've kept one before your doctor starts these tests. The doctor will put you through a series of tests:

(a) *Pulp pinch:* This exercise measures the strength in your fin-gers. The doctor will ask you to squeeze a meter as hard as you can in different directions.

(b) *Tinel's sign:* This touch test indicates possible nerve compression or irritation. The doctor will tap on certain spots on your elbow or palm side of your wrist to see if you feel any tingling.

(c) *Finklestein's sign:* This tests for deQuervain's disease. Your doctor will ask you to make a fist with your thumb inside the fist. He or she will then bend your hand down gently but firmly and ask if it hurts.

(d) *Grip strength:* The doctor will probably also have you squeeze an instrument that measures the strength in both hands.

(e) *Wrist flexion test:* This is a simple but telling sign of RSI. The doctor will ask you to bend your wrist down and back. The normal wrist should be able to bend seventy to ninety degrees both ways. Most RSI patients can barely bend or flex their wrists.

(f) *Weber two-point discrimination test:* This tests for light-touch sensibility. The doctor will ask you to close your eyes as he or she touches your fingertips using a wheel-like instrument with blunt spokes and then ask if you feel one or two points. As the intervals between the spokes get closer, it will be harder for you to discriminate whether there are one or two points.

Tell the doctor or technician if any of these tests cause discomfort or pain. It is important that they have this feedback in order to diagnose you properly. You need to be an active participant while being tested. Also, you can ask for a rest break any time during testing. You are injured. These seemingly benign tests may wear you out quickly. But you are the only one who knows when you are tired. So speak up!

• **Other tests:** Your doctor may want to give you another test for nerve compression in addition to the Weber two-point discrimination test. Either he will order an electromyography (EMG) or do a simple Semmes–Weinstein monofilament test, which is less intrusive than the EMG. He also may want to check for arthritis or bursitis.

(a) *Semmes–Weinstein monofilament test:* This is an inexpensive, painless, and easy way to test for nerve damage. The doctor uses what looks like a long, stiff thread or filament or a bristle from a paintbrush. You will be asked to close your eyes once again as the doctor touches various points on your fingers, palm, and wrist. You will simply say yes when you feel something. The doctor may order a nerve conduction electromyography (EMG) to verify his results or he may be satisfied with this test.

(b) *Range of motion:* Besides the wrist, the doctor will ask you to move your arm from your shoulder in a circular movement and at various angles. Most RSI patients have difficulty raising their arms at all.

(c) *Phalen's maneuver* is one of the first tests for diagnosing carpal tunnel syndrome. You will be asked to put your hands together, back to back with fingers pointing toward the floor. If your fingers go numb after a few minutes or get tingly, it means other tests are necessary to confirm the carpal tunnel syndrome diagnosis.

(d) *The EMG or electromyography* is a test that determines the nerve conduction velocity and the extent of any nerve damage you might have. There are two parts of the EMG. In the first part of the EMG, the doctor or lab technician will wrap a cuff around your wrist that acts as a safety grounding wire. Two small electrodes are taped to your finger and palm. These are stimulated with about five separate electrical pulses, which feel like mild electrical shocks. The pulses become progressively stronger. Later, two coils replace the electrodes and the process is repeated.

The second part of this test is the needle EMG, which records normal electrical activity within the muscle itself. Again, the doctor will tape an electrode, slightly larger this time, to the top of your wrist and insert the tip of a needle along certain muscles. The doctor will ask you to push or pull on your arm during the test while he records it.

Do not use any creams or lotions before taking the tests as they can interfere with the results. Also, cold can obstruct proper interpretation of the test findings. Therefore, the doctor may ask you to warm your hands under water before beginning. An EMG can be quite painful, ranging from discomfort to sharp pain, depending on the severity of your RSI. Relaxation is the key to minimizing the pain during this test. Anxiety only worsens the pain. It is important that your doctor take the entire clinical examination into account before the final diagnosis is made since there are often borderline findings from an EMG.

(e) *The MRI:* In some instances, your doctor may order a *magnetic resonance imaging test* (MRI), which is basically a fancy X ray that offers an important perspective on your joints and muscles. The receptionist will schedule you to go to a different facility for your MRI. For the MRI your shoulders or arm or upper torso—depending on which part of your body is to be imaged—slide into a tunnel-like chamber. When the actual X ray begins, you will hear a loud knocking noise. The procedure doesn't hurt but some of my patients have said that the experience is slightly claustrophobic. The good news is that an MRI lasts only thirty to forty minutes and the image can reveal to your doctor problems not only in bone but in muscles and tendons as well. As a result, the MRI can detect arthritis, bursitis, and rheumatism and is invaluable.

Discovering Underlying Problems

There are other conditions, as we mentioned before, that mask or complicate the diagnosis of RSI. It is necessary to diagnose and treat any underlying causes of pain before starting treatment for what may seem to be the pain from RSI. For example, if the pain you are experiencing is caused by thyroid disease, treating the thyroid condition with medication will remove the pain.

Nathan was a fifty-one-year-old newspaper editor when his arms and hands began to ache and tingle. He thought this was RSI since he had recently seen many of his coworkers diagnosed and treated for the condition. Like many RSI sufferers, Nathan let his pain go untreated for six months, hoping it would go away. Finally, he scheduled a doctor's visit and was tested for various kinds of RSI but all the results were negative. At that point, he read about associated conditions and asked to be tested for thyroid disease and diabetes. Further testing showed that Nathan had very early symptoms of adult diabetes. His doctor immediately put him on a strict diet and gave him appropriate medication for his condition. After a few weeks, the pain and discomfort in his arms went away completely.

Another patient, Mary, who was pregnant, complained of sharp, shooting pain in her hands and arms. She told me that she had no discomfort before she was pregnant. After a thorough examination, I diagnosed her with carpal tunnel syndrome. But her prognosis was good; many pregnant women develop symptoms of CTS but have their symptoms completely disappear once their babies are born. Water retention, hormonal changes, and undue stress as the woman's body changes to accommodate the growing fetus may strain the median nerve and swell the carpal tunnel region. This was the case for Mary's CTS. Soon after she had a beautiful baby boy, the pain in her arms disappeared.

Conditions That May Predispose a Person to RSI

Some diseases, drugs, double-jointedness, age, and lifelong habits can put you at a higher risk for RSI. If you recognize one or more of these conditions and you also have pain, numbness, or tingling in your hands or arms, you should definitely see a doctor immediately. Diseases that may increase the chance of RSI are alcoholism, obesity, rheumatoid arthritis and osteoarthritis, kidney and thyroid disease, and gout. Certain prescription drugs cause water retention and swelling of soft tissues leading to nerve compression problems such as cubital tunnel syndrome. Double-jointedness can also make one more vulnerable to RSI as it causes the joints to collapse when pushed. When the hands, fingers, and wrists are bent thousands of times daily, severe strain can result.

Age is not a factor by itself. However, RSI is, as we noted, a cumulative injury. So the longer you work, the higher your risk is for RSI. Five years ago, when the first book on RSI came out, the average age of the RSI sufferer was thirty-nine. But computers are now typically introduced to children in grammar schools, much sooner than they used to be. As a result, today more and more college students are being diagnosed with RSI.

Unfortunately in the United States, grammar-school-age children are not being trained in the benefits of ergonomics and RSI prevention. Therefore, I think we will see a trend of younger people being injured at a higher rate. France has already started to educate and protect its young. Primary-school children are being taught how to sit in front of a computer at their desks with minimum strain, how to use a keyboard safely, and how to best lift and carry book bags that often weigh forty pounds. With this kind of simple instruction, millions will avoid the pain and slow healing process of RSI. We hope the United States will take this obvious cue and institute a similar program. Until then, parents should take the initiative to protect their children's health by sharing information on RSI prevention through proper posture, rest breaks, and deep-breathing practices.

More Women than Men?

There is a vast difference between the way men and women approach their health care, which puts men at a high risk for RSI. Statistically, male patients account for only 40 percent of physicians' visits. Seventy-eight percent of American women have had a health exam in the last twelve months compared to only 60 percent of American men. Various theories abound as to why there is such a discrepancy in the United States. Men, for example, are afraid of appearing dependent and vulnerable while women, traditionally the caregivers for children and the elderly, are more sophisticated medical consumers. Men tend to ask fewer questions about prognosis, treatment, side effects, and sexuality in order to make informed decisions about their health. Men tend to short-change themselves by being what they view as the "good patient"—one who is quiet and more willing to give up control. These passive habits may make men easier to treat but it doesn't necessarily serve them well.

RSI strikes an equal amount of men and women but, for a while, there seemed to be a higher number of women *reporting* RSI injuries than men. With computer technology creating tighter deadlines and computer use increasing, men are becoming equally vulnerable to the

---

THE DIFFERENCE BETWEEN FINE AND GROSS MOTOR MOVEMENT

Fine motor movement involves short defined strokes with the emphasis on small muscle groups. Writing, typing, drawing, punching a cash register, tapping, designing, decorating a cake—all are fine motor movements. When done repetitively, the smaller muscles used in these movements wear down, fray, and RSI sets in.

Gross motor movement involves movement using mostly the larger muscle groups. Activities such as walking, swimming, dancing, and stretching are all gross motor movements.

It's a good idea to use fine and gross movements alternately when working at any task. Varying your movements will diminish your chances of getting RSI.

---

injury. However, it seems that it is more acceptable for a woman to tend to her injury than for a man. As RSI is better understood and known by the public, I believe more men will consider the discomfort and pain serious before they are disabled by it.

Factors That Can Increase the Chances of RSI and Heighten Its Symptoms

In many studies, patients report that weather changes greatly aggravate their RSI. Cold or humid weather often causes increased pain and discomfort. A lack of sleep or restless sleep, poor nutrition, and sedentary lifestyles are all factors that can also increase the amount of pain associated with RSI. An *overly* physically active lifestyle, such as regularly working double shifts on an assembly line, then going home to cook and clean house, allows your muscles no chance to rest and recuperate and can increase your risk of RSI.

What to Do?

Keep warm and keep moving. Cold sensitivity is often the result of diminished circulation from compression of the arteries and swelling. Activities that use the whole body and big muscles like walking, yoga, or warm-water aerobics as well as full-body gentle exercise of any kind will help increase circulation and decrease the pain. (See chapter 5 on walking, chapter 7 on yoga, and chapter 8 on exercise.)

If you live in a cooler climate, keep a pair of gloves, a scarf, and a sweater handy that you can wear inside as well as out. Often offices are kept at a cool temperature to keep computers operating at their best. So, you may want to adopt these measures even in warmer regions if you work in an air-conditioned building. Silk glove liners are a good substitute if all your gloves feel too tight or heavy. These liners are loose and insulate the hands quite well indoors as well as outside. (See the appendices for ordering information.)

So, now you know what will happen once you arrive at the doctor's office and you have learned about some secondary conditions to discuss with your physician. But how do you choose the doctor who is right for you? What questions should you ask during your first session with your doctor and/or physical therapist? If you are going for a second opinion or looking for a specialist, how do you know the referral is suitable for you?

Choosing Your Doctor

Your primary-care physician coordinates your treatment. He or she is your *home base* and will usually keep the broad picture of your recovery in mind regardless of the changes you go through or the various treatments and therapies you experience on your road back to health. As a general rule, you will exchange ideas with, listen to, and ask the most questions of this doctor.

Sometimes the doctor who diagnoses you is not the best physician for your treatment. A doctor can be a top-notch diagnostician without being connected to any adequate physical therapy facility. I always encourage my patients to *shop* for the right health provider. By this I simply mean for them to look for a doctor who listens and communicates well. Other patients can be the best source of information when you are shopping for a physician.

Once you have met with your candidate for primary-care physician, you will probably notice good and bad points about your first meeting. Think of it as a first date. You need to meet with this person more than

---

QUESTIONS TO ASK FELLOW RSI SUFFERERS
ABOUT DOCTORS THEY RECOMMEND

- **What is the doctor's specialty or area of expertise?** Always cross-check answers you receive from friends or fellow RSI sufferers with the doctor you plan to see since people sometimes fit their answers to what they need. The doctor they suggest may be great for them but not have the specialty you are looking for.
- **What were your expectations?** Remember, everyone's needs are different. Your expectations may be quite dissimilar to those of other patients.
- **What was the reason for seeking this doctor's care?** This should elicit a wealth of information that should help you determine whether or not this doctor will be appropriate for you.
- **Did the doctor listen attentively to you?** A physician who doesn't listen well won't be able to work in a partnership with you. There needs to be a give-and-take of information between you and your doctor. At this point, it might be wise to note how the other patient communicates. Does he or she talk non-stop? Does he or she listen well? These observations will help you interpret the answers you hear.
- **Did the doctor clearly explain your condition and recommend treatment?**
- **Did you feel the doctor charged fairly for his or her time?** It's always important to consider your finances. Check with your insurance company and make sure the doctor you plan to visit will be covered.

---

once to really develop a working relationship. The first few *dates* establish whether or not you believe you can work together. I suggest you consider the following points before making your final choice:

- **Did this doctor answer all your questions adequately?** Remember that good communication takes time and work from both parties. But if a doctor does not answer your questions to your satisfaction, this should be an immediate red flag.
- **Does your doctor follow up on all your concerns?** Two scenarios usually occur: Old and new issues are answered to your satisfaction, or old concerns are addressed to your satisfaction but new concerns are triggered when you reach home. Write them down and follow up on your next visit. If your doctor does not answer your continuing questions, you

may want to look for a different primary health provider. You have to trust your doctor and feel that he or she will listen and follow up on any concerns you have.

• **Are you airing all the questions you have?** Do you feel comfortable asking questions of your doctor? If not, why not? Is it his or her manner or yours? Are you usually shy? Do you think it's rude to ask questions? Do you need to bring a friend along to your next visit to support you and remind you of your questions? Many patients do not get their needs met, not through any fault of the physician but because they are naturally reticent or are afraid to ask anyone health questions. Don't cheat yourself. Ask, and get those questions answered. Knowledge will help you heal faster.

When You Need a Second Opinion

Patients look for second opinions for a variety of reasons, all of which are valid. Sometimes the chemistry isn't right between doctor and patient. Sometimes the patient feels a need for validation of the first diagnosis. And sometimes the patient is looking for other treatment options along with a more hopeful prognosis. Doctors are in the business of helping heal people so if another opinion can help that process so much the better. I am not threatened or insulted if a patient seeks a second opinion. I always encourage it if it will set my patient's mind at ease.

With RSI, second opinions can sometimes mean the difference between living a life of chronic pain with minimal use of the hand or arm and full recovery. Too many doctors still don't believe RSI is a real condition. The educational process among medical professionals concerning musculoskeletal cumulative conditions such as this is slow. However, you shouldn't suffer just because your physician's belief system isn't up-to-date. Many of my patients have come in with horror stories about doctors who didn't believe their accounts of RSI pain and complications. Various patients with clear cases of RSI told me that they are accused of malingering in order to get out of work, told they were hysterical, and called hypochondriacs. If a physician greets you with any of these opinions, keep looking.

When you find a physician with whom you are comfortable, ask him if he has any other patients with RSI. Find out what kind of physician she is and what her specialty is. Physicians, like most human beings, enjoy talking about themselves. By interviewing your doctor, you will also introduce the model of treatment that you hope to embark upon with him or her. You are going to be an active participant in your treatment and your doctor should be open to that. Don't hesitate to get a second opinion if you think your exam is superficial or the doctor seems unwilling or too unfamiliar with RSI, or doesn't seem willing to work *with* you in your recovery.

Once you've received a diagnosis from a doctor you trust, then it's time to look at your treatment options. The next chapter will explore these and discuss actions you can take to help you feel better as soon as possible. Before we move on, let's look at a few points to remember concerning diagnosis.

Points to Remember:

1. Your pain is real. Don't hesitate to seek relief and treatment. See a doctor immediately.
2. Get a diagnosis as soon as you suspect RSI.
3. Make sure your diagnosis is complete. Discuss with your doctor any underlying conditions or diseases that might influence an RSI diagnosis. Schedule the appropriate tests.
4. If you are not satisfied with the diagnosis, seek out a second opinion. Many of my patients have seen three or four physicians before coming to me. RSI is not a widely understood condition by many doctors. Be sure you have one who does understand it and is willing to work with you to treat it.
5. Start a medical journal right away. It will help your diagnosis and treatment plan. Note the kinds of activities you do every day. See if they use the same muscle groups (fine or gross) and similar kinds of movements (small or large, static or repetitive). Show the journal to your chosen physician.

3. Step Two: Develop Your Treatment Plan

After you are diagnosed, your doctor will most likely sit you down and describe his suggested treatment plan, which will usually involve physical therapy, rest, exercise, and, perhaps, occupational therapy or surgery. Physical therapy is usually recommended one to three times a week at first. The doctor may also suggest massage. You can ask to see an occupational therapist if you are having problems opening doors, writing, filing, cooking, or performing other daily activities. The occupational therapist will show you ways to compensate while you are healing.

Your doctor should also give you an idea of your prognosis—how long it will take you to heal and what your chance is for a full recovery. If, for some reason, he doesn't give you a prognosis, ask him about it. Your doctor should reevaluate you every six to eight weeks. If he or she does not mention future visits, bring it up. During these future office visits, he will discuss your progress and adjust your treatment plan. Bring your symptom journal to each office visit.

Your goals in this chapter are to continue developing the partnership between you and your doctor and to begin healing. You should discuss your proposed treatment plan and prognosis with your doctor. Find out what progress you can realistically expect in the next eight weeks, and ask your doctor for suggestions about what you can do on your own to help break the pain cycle of RSI.

The first step in your treatment plan will most likely be a prescription for physical therapy. If your doctor suggests surgery right away, ask about less intrusive therapies first. Then, if physical therapy doesn't alleviate your symptoms, surgery is always an option. If you feel the need for counseling because you are feeling overwhelmed or depressed, this is the time to speak up as well. Your treatment plan needs to suit your needs and it can only do that if you discuss them openly and regularly with your doctor. It also should be revised at each stage of your recovery.

Physical Therapy

The first visit to your physical therapist will be similar to your first doctor's visit in that the physical therapist (PT) will evaluate your range of motion, grip strength, flexibility, and muscle tone. Physical therapy, in general, employs nonintrusive techniques that will help you break your pain cycle and heal. When the evaluation is finished, it's your turn to ask questions such as:

• What kind of training do you have—have you worked with RSI patients before? Have you taken any special courses that might benefit me—learned any alternative techniques that you think might be appropriate?

• How many times will I see you and how long is each session?

• How should I feel after each therapy session? Will I feel achy or tired? Is that normal?

• If I am in pain after the session, what can I do at home to alleviate my discomfort?

• And on the second or third visit: What is your treatment plan for me and when should I expect to feel some improvement?

You may not get answers to all these questions until you have seen the therapist a few times. The PT may need time to work with you and get to know your weaknesses and strengths before he or she will know what alternative methods are appropriate for your case. That's fine. This is a process that will take time as you create a healing partnership.

Because of today's insurance stipulations and sometimes because of your busy schedule, your doctor may start you out with less frequent therapy than is optimum for your recovery. Two times a week is good, three times is often better in severe cases. Ask your doctor why he is suggesting the particular number of sessions. If his answer reflects a motive that is anything other than your quick recovery, you may want to ask him to reconsider his prescription.

Physical therapy can involve very passive to extremely aggressive techniques. Most physical therapy for RSI starts with a passive approach that becomes more active on your part as your condition improves. Passive therapy is still hands-on but the therapist does the work while you relax. She will gently move your injured limbs, stretching and increasing their range of motion. TENS and ultrasound, which I will describe in detail shortly, are two other kinds of passive therapy. More aggressive techniques include deep-tissue massage and various kinds of exercise I will elaborate on as well. As you progress, the therapist will add exercises, weights, and elastic exercise bands (strips of latex that are used as you exercise) to your sessions and recommend you do more exercise on your own as well.

During your diagnosis with the doctor and your evaluation with the therapist, you can begin your education as to which of your muscle groups need exercising and which need extra rest. Your therapist will show you exercise routines you can do at home every day. Muscles heal better when they are allowed to move so practice these routines as often as you can. The exercises will strengthen and tone your muscles as well as increase your overall flexibility and range of motion.

Physical Therapy Techniques Proven
Effective for RSI

There are a variety of techniques your therapist may employ to help you heal. Each technique addresses a different issue such as strengthening, toning, reduction of inflammation, increasing flexibility and range of motion, or reducing sensitivity. I encourage all my patients to ask questions during their physical therapy in order to learn as much as possible about their weaknesses and strengths. The more you understand, the easier it will be not to reinjure yourself. Also, if you know which techniques are for which problem, you can often apply some of these therapies at home and relieve your pain as it arises.

Below are some physical therapy methods that have proven to be especially effective when treating RSI.

Transcutaneous Electrical Nerve Stimulation (TENS)

TENS is basically electronic nerve stimulation. It increases the level of serotonin in the blood, which enhances the effect of natural pain-relieving substances called *endorphins*. This treatment is commonly used to relax muscles. Your therapist will first apply a cool gel to the surface of several electrodes to help them conduct gentle electrical vibrations. Then these battery-generated electrodes, carrying low-voltage electricity, will be placed along pain-ridden areas of your body. You will feel gentle, pleasant vibrations that should reduce pain and allow you to move the treated limb more freely. Home TENS units are available. Ask your therapist whether or not a home unit would be appropriate for you.

TENS therapy is usually harmless but can have adverse effects if you have or are on the cusp of having reflex sympathetic dystrophy (RSD)—a condition where the autonomic nervous system is believed to shut down creating superficial sensitivity and constant pain. In other words, no matter how light the touch, it is painful. TENS should also not be used if you have a pacemaker. Please check with your doctor if you have either of the above conditions.

Ultrasound with Cortisone Cream

Ultrasound helps reduce inflammation and pain. To give an ultrasound treatment, the therapist applies a conductive gel or cortisone cream on the painful area and then lightly moves a handheld ultrasound device in small circles on your skin. Through the device, the ultrasound generator (a box with switches run by electricity that is brought to the side of the therapy table) emits sound waves that can be pulsed or constant. Pulsed or constant sound waves generate heat, which helps reduce pain and increase the elasticity of scar tissue.

Hot and Cold Packs

Hot packs can relieve chronic pain but also are used in physical therapy to relax muscle groups before deep-tissue massage or other aggressive techniques. The heat they provide will increase the circulation in your injured tissues and loosen any toxic lactic acid buildup so it can be washed away. The physical therapist will place the heat packs on the painful areas of your arms, hands, neck, and shoulders as you lie on the treatment table. The weight as well as the heat forces your muscles to relax, allowing you to move more easily. As with anything in therapy, if the heat becomes uncomfortable, speak up.

Cold packs reduce inflammation and swelling and kill pain. Similar to the hot-pack treatment, the therapist will place cold packs wrapped in towels on your inflamed areas as you lie comfortably on the treatment table. As your tissues cool, the inflammation decreases and you can begin gentle movement exercises. Some of my patients also use cold gel packs at home. Since cold reduces flexibility, allow time for your hands and arms to warm up again before exercising. Either gently massage inflamed areas with the packs or just wrap them around the painful areas. Another way of applying ice therapy at home is by freezing a water-filled paper cup. Rip off a small portion of the top of the paper cup and rub the ice on your inflamed area. When you are finished, put the unused portion back in the freezer. But remember that moderation is the key. *Apply the ice just long enough to numb the area.* Too much ice—or heat—will produce the opposite effect of what you are looking for.

If you have circulatory problems, diabetes, Raynaud's disease, rheumatoid arthritis, or any other condition that makes you especially sensitive to cold, check with your doctor before using ice therapy. Make sure you inform your physical therapist about any of the above conditions.

Heat and cold reduce pain in different ways. Cold reduces inflammation and pain and heat relaxes muscle spasms and cramps allowing you to gently stretch and move. Most of my patients report that *alternating cold and heat therapies is most effective for reducing painful symptoms* at home. For an easy self-treatment, purchase two medium-sized plastic window boxes. Fill one with cold water and one with warm water. Alternately place your hand and forearm in each for about ten to fifteen minutes, ending with the warm water. Be careful that you don't strain your shoulder or neck by standing in an awkward position while you soak your arms. Make sure the height of each window box is comfortable.

Stretching and Warm-ups

Your physical therapist will show you exercises that you can do every morning and evening at home. Ask your PT to give you handouts diagramming each exercise with the dos and don'ts plainly spelled out. You may think you will remember them all, but pain creates stress, which weakens the memory. Pay close attention to the instructions and put these exercises to use daily as advised. It's important to get in the habit of warming up every morning before you begin your day and at night before you sleep. Most of us are stiff first thing in the morning and RSI only makes morning movement that much more difficult. Gentle exercises will get your circulation going again and introduce movement to your body as you start your day. The evening exercises will help ease your tired hands and arms and the more relaxed you are at night, the better, more restful sleep you will have.

As you exercise in physical therapy and at home remember not to hold your breath during any of the treatments or exercise routines. It is important to keep nourishing your system with enough oxygen to enable it to work without stress or strain. Many of my patients tell me that they actually feel their bodies relax after taking a deep breath. Try taking a big breath now and letting it out. Feel the difference in the muscles throughout your body. Our goal is to move as efficiently and easily as possible. Breathing deeply and smoothly is a large part of that effort.

You will learn to pace yourself and manage your pain as you exercise and establish your daily pain-management routine. Some of my patients stretch and use cold and hot packs up to ten times a day—at home, at work, and while traveling. Do as much as you feel comfortable with, but just make sure you are not overdoing it. If you feel good after any treatment at home or with the PT, you are probably okay. When in doubt, discuss your frequency of exercise with your physical therapist.

Released and Tense Muscles

You now know that unnecessary tension in the skeletal muscles sets the stage for numerous ligament and joint injuries such as RSI. Tense muscles eventually lose their flexibility and become more vulnerable to injury. Sitting at your computer with your shoulder muscles hunched or holding your arms up while you punch the keys on a cash register are all repetitive stress activities that can contribute to RSI. Massage and physical therapy focus on these static muscles, working to unglue, stretch, and relax tissues and muscle groups.

Released muscles are those that *work only as much as needed in order to perform a particular task. Tense muscles,* on the other hand, *do more work than is necessary.* Released muscles work efficiently; tense muscles work inefficiently. Releasing muscles is a skill. That's why you need to learn specific exercises from your physical therapist. Massage therapy reinforces the relaxation and helps it along. By correcting how we hold and use our heads, necks, and torsos most of the stress in our bodies vanishes. This allows us to carry out our daily activities efficiently. You probably were injured because you used these elements of your body in a stressful and inefficient way.

A *word of caution:* If you hurt while you are doing the exercises at home, there is a good chance you are doing too much or you are doing them incorrectly. Don't just plow ahead. Substitute some gentle stretches until you can practice the exercises in front of your therapist and be corrected. A frequent complaint I hear is, "But my physical therapist told me I had to do these exercises!" Your PT is not omniscient. Remember to use your common sense.

Massage

Massage therapy has been successfully coupled with physical therapy in most of my RSI patients' treatment. In my experience, the earlier massage is introduced, the speedier your recovery is likely to be. Sometimes a good massage may be more helpful than any rigorous exercise routine. However, some PTs don't use massage. If you feel you might benefit from a massage, ask your doctor for a referral. Some insurance plans are even beginning to cover medical massages. Massage is becoming more popular as its positive effects on RSI and other ailments are noted. In fact, the *New England Journal of Medicine* reported in 1993 that massage is the third most used form of alternative medicine in the United States.

Massage also helps our bodies regain their natural alignment. Massage releases the muscles in the neck, at the base of your skull, and at the upper spine, allowing your body to naturally align itself. This reduces the stress and pressure on the neck caused by poor posture and awkward positioning, stress and pressure that can constrict muscles and nerves and lead to RSI. A good massage often offers relief from pain symptoms resulting from muscle spasms, tendinitis, muscle fatigue, inflammation, and swelling.

Massage can also reduce the toxic fluid accumulation and swelling around an RSI injury. It stimulates blood circulation through the veins and lymphatic vessels, which also improves the oxygen flow to all parts of the body and relaxes the muscles that are in tight spasm. With these benefits comes increased flexibility and range of motion and a decrease in pain. Besides being an excellent addition to your general pain-management program, massage can also contribute to your overall feeling of emotional well-being, which can, in turn, increase your quality of life and speed your recovery.

When looking for a massage therapist, make sure the ones you call or visit are licensed by the American Massage Therapy Association. This organization has over forty thousand members and has helped establish licensing laws and standards that are used nationally. When you interview therapists or meet the one your doctor referred you to for the first time, ask if they have experience with RSI. You may have to experiment with a few different therapists before you find the right fit for you. If your doctor doesn't have any suggestions on whom to see for massage, or if you simply want more than one from which to choose, you can network with other RSI patients and ask about their experiences with massage therapists in your area.

Mark Schmetterer, a Manhattan-based massage therapist who has worked with hundreds of RSI patients, suggests that there are a few important aspects to a "good" massage. He believes that the therapist's attention and touch during the massage is as important as the massage technique and that the patient's ability to relax during a massage is just as important as the cleansing and increased mobility a treatment provides. He told me, "It's rare that someone doesn't respond to massage. Even ten minutes of work on the upper back and neck areas can release the tension and pinching that starts to take place with RSI. When you relax the body, it facilitates the carrying away of the waste products and prevents toxic buildup. Massage, like physical therapy, also provides a break for most people when they can't do anything except relax. Most of my patients are on the run and really benefit from this imposed rest period. And many are responsible for families, jobs, you name it. Massage is a time when they are cared for. We all need a moment when we can relax and heal with no other demands made on us."

Massage Techniques and RSI

There are a variety of massage techniques that can benefit you as you recover from RSI. Different techniques work for different people. However, the following types of massage have been especially effective for my patients. Ask your massage therapist with what approach he or she intends to begin and why. A therapist will probably try different techniques as he or she comes to know your body and its condition and as your needs change with time.

• **Medical massage** is prescribed by a doctor and focuses on specific muscle groups. It is different from other kinds of massage in that the therapists who practice it have a thorough understanding of biome-chanics (how the body functions). As a result of this knowledge, he or she may work on your neck or thoracic region and you may feel relief in your hands and arms. In a good medical massage, the strokes are gentle and go only as deep as you can tolerate. This kind of massage is espe-cially good for those with RSI as it concentrates on releasing specific muscle groups that can change *how* you move, allowing you a wider range of movement and flexibility. Explaining how you believe your RSI occurred will help the therapist plan which areas to concentrate on dur-ing your treatment—so speak up!

• **Soft-tissue manipulation and myofascial release:** *Soft-tissue manip-ulation* is a style of massage that usually focuses on the release of muscles and the connective tissues around the spine. The therapist will often combine deep pressure, stretching, and traction techniques. The goal of this massage is to relax the muscles in your neck and back and to move the fluids in order to reestablish circulation and remove toxic wastes.

Myofascial release is the loosening of fixed connective tissues around the muscles through deep manipulation of both the muscles and fascia. This technique has been successfully combined with TENS for even better results. During this kind of body work/massage, the therapist applies the TENS along acupuncture points or painful areas of the body. As I mentioned before in my more detailed discussion of TENS, you will feel a pleasant buzzing when the machine is turned on and increased relaxation as the treatment continues. Some pain centers use stronger TENS vibrations not only to relax but to exhaust the muscles. Then, when the therapist begins the actual massage, the muscles are so tired that they don't contract when touched. This allows the therapist to go deeper with a massage and release locked muscles and glued tissues to a greater degree.

These techniques are just a few kinds of body work and massage that work well for RSI recovery. Other techniques are discussed in chapter 9 where we address the issues of pain management in greater detail. As you seek treatment from massage therapists, remember that if you feel your RSI symptoms are not improving ask your doctor for his/her advice. Your health is the primary concern. If something doesn't work, perhaps you can resolve it and you should always feel free to find a new person with whom to work.

You have already begun to participate in your treatment program by asking questions of your doctor, physical and massage therapists, and by practicing home exercises. The next step is to learn how to breathe correctly while you move.

4. Step Three: Take a Deep Breath

Place one hand on your chest and one hand on your belly. Breathe normally for a few moments, noticing which hand moves as you inhale. Which rises the most? If it's the one on your stomach, pat yourself on the back. You have excellent respiratory technique. If the hand on your chest rises higher, you need to focus and practice breathing from your diaphragm. Not only will deep diaphragmatic breathing help your RSI, it will also give you the added bonus of more energy for all you do. You'll be happy to hear that you can access this reservoir of extra energy with just a little effort.

The goal of this chapter is to help you enjoy a whole new world full of relaxation and peace. Many of my patients tell me they have fewer painful flare-ups and can move more comfortably after mastering diaphragmatic breathing and the relaxation response. These techniques are an invaluable help to an RSI treatment plan. I've found that, following their recovery, many patients continue to practice both methods of relaxation as a kind of meditative reminder of how to stay healthy and relaxed.

How we breathe influences every part of our physical and emotional health. In chapter 1 we covered why oxygen debt is one of the major physical causes of RSI. If you are a chest breather, as too many of us are, the oxygen molecules you inhale remain in your upper lungs and don't diffuse into a large proportion of your blood vessels, which are most intensively concentrated in the lower lobes of the lungs. If oxygen doesn't get to all the blood vessels in the lower lungs, the muscles and organs that are waiting for it throughout your body can be underoxygenated. Your muscles need all the help they can get to relax while you move especially if you suffer from RSI. Oxygen is the key to this dynamic.

Chest breathers have to breathe faster than diaphragm breathers to get enough oxygen. That's where the trouble begins. Exhaling carbon dioxide too quickly, as chest breathers are apt to do in their quest for more oxygen, disturbs the balance of acidity and alkalinity—known as pH—in the blood. When the acid levels drop, a complex reaction occurs that actually keeps the blood cells from delivering oxygen to all the body's muscles and organs. The end result is hyperventilation. Stress, anxiety, and exercising too hard are only a few triggers of hyperventilation, which, in extreme cases, can cause you to get dizzy or even pass out. If you breathe from your chest, a lower-level hyperventilation can take place during every breath you take, every day.

But what does all this have to do with RSI? Many of us are in the habit of holding our breath whenever we concentrate. Our breath often becomes shallow until we finish a movement or complete a thought. This habit strains our muscles. Because we are not breathing properly, we are not circulating away the waste products the way we should be, which allows the toxic lactic acid to build up. Breathing is an important aspect of the circulation and cleansing processes. The oxygen in our blood not only energizes muscles but also helps remove the unwanted waste. You can see that if we don't breathe deeply, our muscles are adversely affected, which makes each and every motion more taxing for us.

Therefore, one of the first things your muscles must be trained to do when you have RSI is to *move while relaxing*. To do so, you must learn how to breathe properly. The more oxygen you can feed your muscles when you are moving, the more relaxed you will be and the sooner you will heal. So, if you want to feel better, stop holding your breath.

I always know a physical therapist is good if one of the first exercises my patients report learning is one that illustrates how to breathe correctly while exercising. It simply involves taking three slow deep breaths, with arms comfortably at one's side *before* beginning the exercises. This accomplishes two things: It warms up the muscles and relaxes them so they are ready to move without strain.

If you practice deep diaphragmatic breathing on a regular basis, which is what you are doing when you follow this exercise, you will begin to breathe better regularly. You may not be able to totally overhaul your respiratory style and breathe deeply all of the time, but learning to slow your ventilation with periodic diaphragmatic breathing throughout your day can short-circuit your body's response to stress.

How to Practice Diaphragmatic Breathing

Lie on your back with one hand on your abdomen. Start by inhaling through your nose, filling the abdominal region (your hand should rise). Continue to inhale to fill your rib cage and finally your upper chest. Hold that breath for one second and then exhale slowly through your mouth, allowing your abdomen, rib cage, and upper chest to empty in a wavelike motion. Take a second or two to rest before inhaling again. This is called *complete breath* by some, and a *three-part breath* by others. Whatever you wish to label it, it is an effective, relaxing way to breathe. Try for an even, comfortable ten seconds of inhalation and a steady ten seconds of exhalation. Repeat three times.

Note: Take the time before you begin this breathing exercise to position pillows around and under you so that you can lie stretched out, relaxed, and without pain. Some of my patients use up to six pillows to support themselves in comfort. Make sure you give yourself this time to be pain free and comfortable.

After you have mastered this technique while lying down, try it in a comfortable sitting position, still touching your abdomen with your hand so you can feel it rise as you inhale. I suggest you begin practicing this technique at least once in the morning and once at night before going to sleep. Don't be surprised if this relaxing practice is one you keep long after the pain of your RSI is gone. Many of my patients tell me the benefits this deep breathing provides are so obvious and comforting that they make this a long-term practice.

Many patients tell me this little habit is also of great help during the day when they are engaged in an activity that suddenly causes pain. They stop, get comfortable, and breathe. I suggest you do the same. The benefits are almost instantaneous.

Note how you feel before and after your breathing exercises in your symptom journal.

For the first week of your daily breathing exercises, jot down how you feel in your journal. As you gradually incorporate these breathing techniques into your exercise routines, note whether your exercises—especially the more strenuous ones—are easier with the new method of breathing.

Also, note how you feel after a cycle of deep breaths upon awakening with pain in the middle of the night. Does it relax you? Does the pain lessen or disappear? Do you prefer to practice the technique lying down or sitting? Discuss your notes with your physical therapist and doctor. They may have valuable feedback for you concerning how your RSI is progressing and how you can adapt to minimize your symptoms while practicing your breathing.

Moderation Is the Key

Until you retrain your muscles to move without strain, it is of paramount importance to slow down while you move so you can move efficiently and without strain. Diaphragmatic breathing slows down your whole system. But many of my patients report that they find it extremely difficult to sit quietly and breathe. Their schedules and fast metabolisms often are not conducive to learning this subtle skill. If you find sitting and breathing difficult, build your technique slowly. Don't add to your frustration and depression by setting unrealistic goals for yourself on this or any other exercise. Just remember: Everyone can learn to breathe quietly and deeply and it does decrease pain. While it may be difficult to do nothing but breathe for a few minutes, it is worth the time and emotional investment. Every deep breath you take will help you move in a healthier and safer way.

I have written many prescriptions for basic yoga because it not only reinforces the lesson of deep breathing but it also teaches my patients to listen to their bodies. It often helps them to heighten their awareness of how they move and, in general, to slow down when they move. Recovering from RSI involves an enormous amount of muscle training. In order to retrain the muscles, the patient has to think about how he moved before and after he was injured. Pushing through pain won't help recovery. Deep breathing and yoga, which increase body awareness and relaxation, are a wonderful help in retraining minds and muscles to slow down and move carefully.

The Mechanics of Stress

When you are stressed, your heart rate speeds up and your blood pressure soars to transport fuel in the form of glucose and oxygen to the muscles. You may perspire and your muscle tone changes. You are getting ready for the very basic fight-or-flight response. You start breathing faster in order to expel the carbon dioxide that's created when the glucose and oxygen are metabolized by your muscles.

This stress response is the same whether your current threat is real or just imagined, and it lowers the effectiveness of the body's mechanisms of self-repair. If this response is extended over a lengthy period of time, stress-related conditions such as bronchial asthma, fatigue, hypertension, nervousness, or insomnia can plague you. In addition, if you become fatigued enough, your posture may change during your work task straining your muscles every time you move. Combine that with your shallow breathing and the result is various kinds of RSI.

When you have deadlines to meet, have to speak at an important luncheon, or are late and stuck in traffic, you get stressed from the same heart racing and quickened respiration of the *sympathetic nervous system* that is responsible for the physiological overdrive that triggers stress. The lucky aspect of the fight-or-flight response is that all of the elements in this reaction—racing heart, rapid breath, sweaty palms—are linked to each other. So if you change one of the responses, such as breathing, they all change. Most of our everyday situations don't generate the full-blown fight-or-flight response, but you can reduce the effect stressful situations have on your body. If you change one easy response when you're rushed or working hard, you can calm down your whole system. All you have to do is take a deep breath.

Controlling Your Respiration

When patients learn to take deep inhalations of air, they report that much of their physical tension melts away and their pain from RSI lessens immediately. This is because when your muscles are getting enough oxygen, they will spasm less, your pain will decrease, and your feeling of well-being will improve. Many stress-reduction clinics, such as the Stress Reduction Clinic at the University of Massachusetts Medical Center in Worcester where more than 10,000 patients have been treated for pain and symptoms related to a wide range of complaints, are strong advocates of deep breathing as stress and pain reducers.

Respiration is both voluntary and involuntary. You breathe all the time without a second thought, but you can consciously alter your respiration style if you want to—or stop it altogether—for brief periods. So if you can learn to breathe deeply, you are on your way to moving without strain, stress, or pain.

The Relaxation Response

Pain is one of the loudest signals for help your body can send. If you are in pain, you need to learn how to listen. To do that, you *must* slow down, rest, relax while you move, and breathe deeply.

In addition to diaphragmatic breathing, there is another technique for controlling your breath that has deep relaxation benefits. Called the *relaxation response*, it is one of the most successful stress relievers for those with RSI. Most of my RSI patients complain of depression, frustration, and anger as well as extreme stress while recovering. I highly recommend this technique to help you address all these RSI symptoms—psychological and physical.

Dr. Herbert Benson discovered the relaxation response, a process that allows you to push aside stressful, intrusive thoughts and focus on repeating a word, sound, prayer, phrase, or muscular activity. This simple practice produces a short-term calming effect on the body. Metabolism, blood pressure, heart rate, rate of breathing, and muscle tension all decrease. The relaxation response gives the body permission to relax. It helps to counter the cumulative effects of stress. I totally concur with Dr. Benson when he tells us we all should pursue good nutrition, exercise, and stress management and make them part of our daily routine. Preventing stressful conditions from developing is one of the main changes all RSI sufferers need to make. The relaxation response will raise your awareness of harmful activities and help you control your stress. It will also heighten your belief in your ability to help yourself get well.

RSI is not usually mentioned when listing conditions that directly benefit from a patient's belief in his power to help himself heal. But I believe it should be. Because of our unconscious muscular-skeletal habits, we accumulate the strains that produce the various kinds of RSI. The more conscious we can make these habits, the easier it is to change them and recover.

To produce the relaxation response you need to repeat a word, a sound, a phrase, or muscular activity. Walking is a perfect repetitive muscular activity that creates no strain for those with RSI. Or repeating the phrase "deep and easy" as you relax. When everyday thoughts intrude on your focus, you have to passively disregard them and return to your repetition. One of my patients, Noah, described the process beautifully: "My time to relax is precious to me, but it usually takes a while before it happens. All the hustle and bustle of my day usually intrudes at first—lists of things to do, the doctor I need to call, my car that needs fixing, food for dinner—but I visualize a shelf where I put all those intruding thoughts. There they wait, not forgotten but put aside as I replace them with my mantra [repeated phrase], and I suddenly find myself sinking into this wonderful relaxed state." The relaxation response can be elicited from a wide variety of techniques including meditation, yoga, tai chi chu'an, prayer, or a walk. You will feel your muscles gradually relax as you get deeper and deeper into the response.

I find it helpful to introduce patients to diaphragmatic breathing first and then practice the relaxation response with them. Learning to breathe correctly also teaches us how to focus. And, as I said before, it begins to slow us down. I have found that as my patients introduce the relaxation response into the daily routine, they begin to move without strain, some of their depression lifts, and the motivation to continue to use the techniques increases.

You are on your way to recovery. You have begun to give your strained muscles enough oxygen, you are learning to reward yourself with relaxation and moderation, and you're incorporating special exercises from physical therapy into your daily routine. You are doing great so far. The next step will help you reduce your symptoms even more and increase your muscle tone and strength. Many of my patients have learned to go for a walk any time the pain becomes overwhelming. Many have finally learned to integrate walking into their daily activities even when the pain is only moderate. Let's find out why it is so important for you to do the same and how you can get started on your walking routine.

5. Step Four: Walk Off Your RSI

Pull on your windbreaker and let's head out the door. You probably don't feel like doing anything. You are in pain and you are most likely depressed. This is one instance when you shouldn't listen to your inner voice. The solution is very simple: WALK. Don't try to figure out how to feel better. JUST WALK.

It doesn't matter where you live or whether it is raining or sunny. If you are in pain, walking will help relieve your symptoms and your depression will begin to dissipate. Get your circulation going. Distract yourself from your pain and MOVE!

The large muscle movements involved in walking relax your more vulnerable muscles injured from RSI. As you walk, your circulation increases, your depression lifts, and your pain temporarily abates. Walking is the first therapy you can do for yourself. You don't need a prescription. You don't need advice. If your hand, wrist, arms, shoulders, or neck begins to hurt, get up and walk. If you feel stiff or your limbs feel heavy and tingle, walk.

If you can find a warm-water pool (80°F or above), walking in a pool will also help tone and maintain your muscle strength without the slight jarring you may experience on land. Water cushions your body and is buoyant, which allows you to move with less stress and strain. But land walking is also extremely beneficial as a stress reliever and pain reducer. You should walk—in water or out—every day.

Your Step Four Goal

Your goal in step four will be to walk forty-five minutes every day. Build up to the forty-five-minute walk slowly if it feels like too much at first. You don't want to become so fatigued or discouraged that you give up before you can reap the benefits. Everything in moderation. Begin with a thirty-minute walk on Tuesday, Thursday, and Sunday. Soon you'll notice that you're walking farther and that it's enjoyable! When the three days feel fundamental, like a part of your routine, naturally add Monday, Wednesday, and Saturday and increase the duration by fifteen minutes. Practice walking into relaxation through an imaginary door. Leave all your pain and troubles behind you.

HOW TO KEEP YOUR WALK INTERESTING

Try these different ideas to introduce variety into your exercise routine.

- **Break out of your routine and take off.** Walk to a museum instead of getting on that bus that aggravates your RSI anyway. Investigate new parks and seek out new terrain in your city or town.
- **Sign up for walkathons.**
- **Walk to socialize.** Walk with a buddy, spouse, or group. Besides being more fun, many find walking with someone on a regular basis an easier way to keep their commitment to walk.
- **If it rains, break out the foul-weather gear.** There are some inexpensive light-weight ponchos that are pain free to wear for RSI sufferers. Or walk around a mall. In many parts of the country there are early mall-walker groups that meet before or after the malls open and use the space like a walking track.
- **Let Mozart accompany you.** If you find music helps you escape and relax, there are wonderful new Walkmans that are light and easy to hang on a belt while taking in the sights on a walk. It's a great time to learn a new piece of music or just enjoy some old chestnuts.

Beating the American Weight Problem

Americans tend to carry around more weight than any other population in the world. We sit too much and, most of the time, we eat too much. When we are anxious and in pain, we tend to eat more. Weight-loss experts claim that walking forty-five minutes daily will help you drop excess pounds and keep them off. If you don't do it, they claim, you probably won't be able to keep weight off no matter what you try.

Melinda, fifty-two, lives in a small town in New York. She wakes up an hour early in order to go to the gym before work. She does a five-minute warm-up on the motorized treadmill and then turns the controls to four miles an hour. While walking she watches the morning news hour. As the credits roll, she knows her workout is over. Like many other professional women, Melinda has no time for fancy planning. Her life is already busy enough. "Walking is a no-brainer. I walk an hour a day. It keeps my weight down as well as being a great cardiovascular workout." As Melinda leaves the gym, she is relaxed and ready for the office. Her muscles are warmed up and ready to work. "As an executive secretary, I have to be very careful about fitness. Using the computer all day puts me at high risk for RSI. Walking is great preventive medicine. And it makes me feel great."

Walking Forty-five Minutes Is Best

The 1996 surgeon general's report recommended thirty minutes of physical activity a day. However, *for RSI relief, a forty-five-minute walk is fundamental to recovery.* When one part of you is injured, it is imperative that you keep the rest of you fit and moving. It takes a good ten minutes to warm up and, at the thirty-minute mark, your circulation should be flowing, your breathing deep and even, and the relaxation response will have kicked in. Then you need at least fifteen more minutes of moving without strain. You also need to practice feeling relaxed. When you've been walking for thirty minutes, your depression will have lessened and you most likely will be enjoying yourself. This may be a new experience for those of you struggling with RSI. In these last fifteen minutes of your walk you retrain your muscles to move efficiently and realize you feel good.

Walking: An Equal Opportunity Benefit

When one part of you is injured, your other uninjured, healthy parts naturally take over the work. Your healthy arm, for example, will do twice to three times the lifting, grasping, pulling, pushing, and twisting movement of your incapacitated limb. This reflexive, compensatory reaction puts your healthy limbs at high risk for overuse and RSI. Walking is the great equalizer. The natural swinging rhythm of walking uses your entire body equally. It redistributes the natural movement and the *work* of moving. It uses your larger muscles, giving your smaller, overused connective tissues the deserved rest they need.

Making Your Daily Walk a Necessity

Many people find that the best intentioned exercise plans easily go unfulfilled. Think of walking in the same way you think of brushing your teeth or washing your face. You would never consider skipping them. Walking should become as fundamental as those other necessities. There is no complex decision to make. Just throw on some sneakers and walk. Whenever you can substitute walking for driving, do so.

Renate, a textile designer in North Carolina, is a perfect model of good planning. She has three friends with severe cases of RSI. They didn't use any preventive techniques in their high-risk jobs. Renate says, "I use the mouse all day to do fabric design on the company's computer. I love my work, but my wrists began hurting after only a week on the job. Now I walk forty-five minutes during my lunch hour. I run my wrists and hands under warm water before I begin work in the morning and after each break. And I do gentle stretches every half hour and then rest for at least ten minutes. I am proud to say that I have the highest quality designs in my company and the largest output." Renate describes walking as her safety net. "I try to walk as much as possible since I have

WALKING IS A MUST FOR THE FOLLOWING PEOPLE:

• Anyone who is diagnosed with RSI or even suspects he is at high risk
• Anyone who sits more than eight hours a day
• Anyone who is outside for less than fifteen minutes per day
• Anyone who experiences joint discomfort when sitting or lying down
• Anyone who experiences tension in his shoulders, neck, or back muscles
• Anyone who considers himself overweight
• Anyone who has a high resting pulse (higher than eighty beats per minute)

PEOPLE WHO SHOULD AVOID WALKING AND CONSULT THEIR PHYSICIAN IMMEDIATELY:

• If you can't walk one hundred yards without experiencing pain
• If your blood pressure is consistently above 140/90 mm Hg.
• If you have an acute infection, fever, or a cold. Acute illnesses have caused lung and heart muscle infections that can be life threatening
• If you have chest pains that change or radiate to the left side of your body
• If you have severe heart irregularity as well as breathing difficulty and chest pain, and severe coronary artery stenosis

As you can see, walking is great for most people. However, to avoid any danger, make sure you get a complete medical examination by your doctor before you start your walking program.

an intense eight hours every day where I just sit. Walking makes me feel better, gives me more energy, and I can actually feel the tension seep out of my muscles after fifteen minutes or so of walking." Most people with RSI don't want to take days off once they start to feel the benefits of walking. But if you must, make up the no-walk day, with an hour-long walk on the days you can exercise.

Pacing Yourself

Walking is a type of endurance sport that gently stimulates the body with the help of oxygen. We breathe at a steady rhythm when we walk, which helps to stabilize excess carbon dioxide and lack of oxygen.

When you exhale, you expel the unwanted carbon dioxide from your body. You are then able to take in oxygen quickly, transferring it via the bloodstream to the muscles, and balance the oxygen debt. If you experience pain or cramping while you walk, it is a sign that your body cannot keep up with the oxygen conversion. If this happens to you, slow down your pace and your rate of breathing. Listen to the signals your body sends out and know your limits. After an hour-long walk, your body may feel pleasantly fatigued but perform less efficiently. This is a signal that you now need rest to regain your normal abilities. The length of your rest depends on your level of physical fitness. When you are breathing easily and your muscles are relaxed you know you can safely resume your walk.

Begin gently, increase slowly. Eventually, you want to reach a comfortable brisk pace when you walk. Walking is a terrific, easy technique since even beginners should immediately feel relief. Pace yourself. The heart, circulatory system, and neuromuscular system adapt much faster to the demands of walking than do other parts of the body such as tendons, ligaments, cartilage, and bones. When you have RSI, your tendons and ligaments are going to adapt more slowly to the demands made on the body during a vigorous walk. Take it easy especially during your first weeks of walking.

Start every walk as if you have someplace to go; focus and move ahead. If you are out of breath, slow down. To find your optimum breathing rhythm, experiment with inhaling three steps and exhaling for the next three steps. If your body needs more oxygen, alternate between inhaling through the nose and mouth. If you try this and are still gasping for air, slow down and then stop. Your goal is to try for at least four miles an hour at a fifteen-minute-per-mile pace, but it may take you some time to get there. Your pace may also be slower or faster than that depending on how long your stride is.

Using Your Target Heart Rate

When you are walking briskly or participating in other vigorous activities, try reaching your target heart rate. Your monitoring of this is simple and is also a good way for you to help health-care professionals to track your progress. As you walk, you need to measure your pulse periodically and stay within 50 to 75 percent of your maximum heart rate. *This range is called your target heart rate.* Each person's rate will differ slightly, depending upon your age, gender, level of fitness, physique, and resting heart rate.

The American Heart Association has developed the table on the following page showing estimated target heart rates for different age categories. Look for the age category closest to yours and read across to find your target heart rate or figure out your target heart rate for yourself with the following equation.

To find your target heart-rate range:

1. Take 220 beats per minute and subtract your age in years. For example: If Joe is forty-five years old, his calculation for this first part is $220 - 45 = 175$.
2. Take 50 percent to 75 percent of the result. Your answer is the target training heart rate, in beats per minute, for you during exercise.

   For example, Joe's target heart rate is between 50 percent of 175, which is 88, and 75 percent of 175, which is 131. If Joe stays within 88 to 131 heartbeats per minute, he is at his ideal heart rate when walking. This is the level at which Joe can comfortably train without undue stress on his heart. This is his optimum range. If his heart rate is faster than this, Joe should slow down. If it is slower, he can safely walk a little faster.
3. To measure your heart rate, find your pulse by applying slight pressure with your fingers (not your thumb, which has its own pulse!) on your wrist on the inside of your forearm. Look at the second hand of your watch and count the heartbeat (pulse) for fifteen seconds. Multiply that number by four and you will have your heart rate per minute.

Frequency and length of your walks will determine your level of stamina and physical comfort when you have RSI. Aim at the lowest part of your target heart-rate zone (50 percent) during the first few weeks. Then gradually build up to the higher end of your target heart-rate zone (75 percent.) If you experience more muscle pain, stiffness,

TARGET HEART RATE FOR MEN AND WOMEN*

Age (years)	Target Heart Rate (beats per minute)	Average Maximum Heart Rate 100%
20 years	100–150 beats per minute	200
25 years	98–146 beats per minute	195
30 years	95–142 beats per minute	190
35 years	93–138 beats per minute	185
40 years	90–135 beats per minute	180
45 years	88–131 beats per minute	175
50 years	85–127 beats per minute	170
55 years	83–123 beats per minute	165
60 years	80–120 beats per minute	160
65 years	78–116 beats per minute	155
70 years	75–113 beats per minute	150

*Although women have smaller hearts and lower heart-blood volume, they do have the same heart rates as men.

tiredness, or exhaustion after you walk, it is a clear signal that you have overtaxed your system. Start slowly and on a sensible schedule. There is no rush.

Note: A few high-blood-pressure medications lower the maximum heart rate and thus the target heart rate. If you are taking high-blood-pressure medicine, contact your doctor to find out if your walking program needs to be adjusted.

The Benefits of Walking for RSI Sufferers

• **Increases stamina.** Exercise increases a person's energy and ability to work and play longer and harder without fatigue. RSI, like any injury, decreases stamina. Walking is an excellent way to keep your stamina high and your whole body toned while you are recovering.

• **Strengthens bones.** The density of bones is controlled mainly by diet, hormones, and exercise. As people get older, bones become thinner and more brittle. Fortunately bones, like muscles, become stronger with use. Weight-bearing exercises such as running and walking are best for keeping bones strong and will prevent the onset, or slow down the progress, of osteoporosis.

• **Helps reduce conditions associated with stress and obesity.** Walking takes your mind off your injury as well as releasing those "happy" endorphins that fight pain and make you feel better. My RSI patients tell me there are too many days when they feel they can do nothing. The answer I always give is walk, walk, walk. Get your system moving again. The pain will decrease. Your depression will lessen. You are actively helping yourself to heal when you walk.

• **Improves diabetes.** Because walking decreases the need for insulin, helps to control weight (a major problem for diabetics), and lowers the risk of cardiovascular disease, it is often prescribed for those with diabetes. Walking is the ideal exercise if you happen to have a combination of diabetes and RSI.

• **Increases strength, flexibility, and balance.** Movement can be limited by 50 percent with some RSI injuries. Walking is a wonderful way to begin to move and flex again. Balance is often a problem when you can't move the way you used to. Walking is safe and will help you reestablish your natural balance and movement. It also releases muscle spasms because you use mostly large muscles thereby relaxing and resting those fine, small muscles that have been injured. Walking increases your circulation, typically pushing five to seven liters (five to seven quarts) of blood through your arteries.

• **Walking lifts depression.** Almost every one of my patients has reported an improvement in mental attitude when he began his walking routine. Spirits lift as depression and anxiety disappear. The National Institute of Mental Health tells us that long-term exercise decreases depression in moderately depressed patients and increases self-esteem in normal people. Some people experience a "walker's high," which some physicians say is the result of the body releasing endorphins. These endorphins cause a sense of well-being. Some scientists think the phenomenon is due to a slight rise in body temperature. Still others feel it has to do with rhythmic exercise.

• **Too much rest is counterproductive.** People in acute pain from RSI often only want to lie down and sleep. This creates problems such as low blood pressure and the deterioration of muscle and bone. A research team at Brooks Air Force Base, under the direction of Dr. Convertino, found that a single bout of exercise can be as effective in reversing these problems as traditional drug treatment.

It is a good idea to pay attention to all of the physical and mental benefits of walking. Ask yourself: How do I feel? Do I feel better? Calmer? Less pain? How am I breathing during this time? When you identify the benefits, it will give you more incentive to walk. And make sure you note your progress in your symptom journal.

Finding the Perfect Balance Between Exercise and Rest

Too much or too little of anything is no good. So how do you find your middle ground between exercise and rest? My patients are constantly struggling with this problem. Professional athletes in sports such as swimming and track and field use a technique called "periodization training." This type of program allows athletes to reach their peak on schedule safely without high risk of overuse and injury. The intensity and frequency of training is controlled. In addition, the athletes are taught how to warm up and cool down and build in rest periods in their training. It might interest you to know that some of the top athletes in the country rest one or two whole days during each week of training. That's twenty-four to forty-eight hours!

A typist who works an average of eight hours a day is an *office athlete*. A truck driver, journalist, surgeon, assembly-line worker—all use their bodies as strenuously and continuously as athletes do. Whatever you do, start thinking of yourself as an athlete. Keep your body limber and strong and your rest periods frequent.

Building Rest into Your Daily Routine

We have to build rest into our daily routine. Muscle tissue needs to pause. Trainers often use the words "rest" and "recovery" interchangeably. Rest refers to doing nothing. Recovery is generally considered to

ATHLETES REST SCHEDULE*

Athlete(s)	Average Days of Rest during Week of Training	Average Rest after an Event or Season
The Knicks *basketball team*	I day	3 to 4 months of rest
Joel McKeever Elaine Asanakis *pairs figure skaters*	2 days	3 to 4 days; I month a year
Lindsay Davenport *tennis player*	I day	After three weeks of play, 3 to 4 days off; I month off a year
Lynne Cox *long-distance swimmer*	I or 2 days	Decreases amount of workout slowly; 6 weeks off a year

*Source: *New York Times*, March 27, 1996

be the period immediately following a workout, when the body adapts to the exercise before it returns to its resting state. Then there is *active rest* where the person participates in activities other than the usual exercise or sport, like walking. In other words, if you sit at a computer all day, your active rest period could be a walk around your building. Another break period could be used to close your eyes and relax for five minutes followed by some gentle warm-up exercises to ready your body for work once again.

The Focused Walk

T. George Harris, editor-in-chief of both *Psychology Today* and *American Health*, collaborated with Lindus Mundy to produce a small guide that offers great insights for those "on the path to body-and-soul fitness." This small guide, available through Abbey Press, describes the benefits of "taking a trip" from the devouring demands of our everyday life. Walk away. Stop the brain commotion and the muscle strains of our constant activities. Research shows that *focused* exercise invokes the relaxation response. Your exercise becomes more efficient as you exercise and simultaneously focus your mind. Focused exercise actually requires less energy to do physical work. This means less strain and stress. At the University of Massachusetts, it was found that focused walking helps reduce anxiety and depression. The repetitive quality of walking helps trigger the relaxation response. Besides toning and flexing your muscles with the gross movements of walking, you are giving your entire sensory system "time off" to relax and reconnect with your inner, more natural rhythms. Focused walking uses the same process as yoga or meditation. When everyday thoughts intrude, you passively dismiss them and return to your repetition, whether it is a sound or the rhythm of your walk. Perhaps you have noticed this response when a baby is put in a mechanical swing or rocked to sleep. The constant rhythm induces relaxation, tunes

WHAT TO WEAR

You may think that clothing is unimportant when you walk, but my coauthor, Ruth, spent a couple of hundred dollars before she found the walking shoe and socks that met her needs. She shares the following observations and research in the hope of helping you.

Walking is a low-maintenance sport. Most of the time, you can just throw on some shorts, a T-shirt, and there you have it. Wear something comfortable that feels good when you walk. Avoid jeans that may be too tight or any top that requires a lot of fussing. Loose T-shirts, sweatshirts, or light sweaters are ideal. Make sure you will be warm enough while you walk but be careful not to get overheated. Remember that you will warm up as your walk progresses.

Shoes

When you hit your feet, it becomes a bit more complicated. You need to make time to find the shoe that fits you. Manufacturers have developed supportive, light, flexible, shock-absorbing shoes to make your walk comfortable. Be particularly picky if you will be mostly walking on asphalt. Shoes that are not exclusively leather can even be washed in a washing machine in warm, not hot, water. Air or gel fillings are particularly good for reducing stress on joints and ligaments. Make sure your shoes are not too small. Let the salesperson or your physician suggest what kind of shoe would fit best with your kind of feet. We all walk differently, turning our feet out or in and have a variety of high or low arches or insteps.

out all the noisy stimuli in our everyday lives. The child takes advantage of this almost hypnotic effect and sleeps. A focused walk, with its repetitive quality of exercise, can dissolve all your stress in the same way—creating the relaxation response.

Getting Back Control

People who walk regularly are more apt to believe they can control what happens to them. They tend to believe in their inner power. In my experience, such people believe that their own motivation has a big impact on their health. When you believe that you have some control over your health, it is much easier to dispel any feeling of helplessness or depression that may result from injuries such as RSI.

Walking magazine and *Consumer's Digest* publish lists of the "Best Shoes/Best Buys" sometimes twice a year. But make sure the shoes you buy are good for *you*. Make sure your toes have enough room and your shoes don't ride up when you take a step. Take a few different thicknesses of socks with you. Some brands may fit fine only with a thinner sock. Look for walking shoes or cross trainers but not running shoes. Find a pair of shoes that have good arch support and thick, flexible soles. Time and money are worth spending for a good shoe that will allow you to walk away your pain.

Socks

When it comes to socks, we usually grab any pair that's clean. But the right socks can protect your feet from moisture, pressure, and irritation. Here are some tips when choosing socks that are designed for fitness walking.

- Look for socks that breathe, socks made from acrylics and other "performance yarns." Cotton, when trapped in a shoe, absorbs moisture and keeps it there. It is not a breathable fabric and can cause blisters when damp.
- Look for socks that provide cushioning on the heels and balls of the feet to prevent shock, abrasion, and fatigue.
- *Walking* magazine (August 1998) recommends specific walking socks from the following manufacturers: Fox River, Wick Dry, Natural Sport, Thorlo, Wigwam, and Brisk. They range from $7.95 to $13.00. (This magazine also has great ideas in each issue about walking adventures you may want to take!)

My patients who exercise regularly usually discover that other parts of their lives become healthier as a result. They begin to be more careful about what they eat, are less likely to smoke and more likely to give up smoking than people who do not exercise. A regular exercise program gives you back some of the control that RSI takes away in other areas of your life. Plan to incorporate one into your daily routine.

Walking is easy, needs no special equipment, and is always available to you. Most of my patients find that once they begin to walk regularly, other changes come more easily. And they feel better. Now let's take a look at how to fuel all this exercise and activity. There are certain foods that benefit healing and some that will trigger more muscle spasms and cramps. Chapter 6 will tell you how to keep your system running at its optimum level of health.

6. Step Five: Create Your RSI Nutrition Plan

This is not intended to be another diet book. I simply want to empha-size some of the specific nutritional dos and don'ts I provide for my RSI patients. When you have RSI, your body needs to have a steady supply of nutrients to mend ligaments, tendons, and muscles. The best and most healthy diet you can maintain is eating foods in as close to their natural state as possible. Processed foods contain all sorts of chemicals and fats that will eventually hurt you. A diet of broiled or baked meats and fish, steamed vegetables, rice and beans, grilled vegetables in olive oil and spices, and potatoes is one that offers nearly everyone variety and health. Make sure you get enough protein and you are giving your body enough "fuel" to heal. The benefits this kind of diet provides a healing body such as yours are invaluable.

Your RSI nutrition plan is designed to:

- Reduce muscle spasms and pain
- Battle depression and/or apathy
- Moderate your weight so it is appropriate to your height and build
- Control inflammation
- Increase energy.

Your body uses nutrients simultaneously to fight injury or for some metabolic response. The nutrients are like links in a chain. The whole chain equals health. If one link is rusty or weak, the entire chain is weakened and may break down. A healthy daily diet builds up the body's store of nutrients over time to develop strong defenses and quick healing properties. Taking one vitamin E every now and then won't cut it. Nutrients are not fast food. Educating yourself about nutrition and designing your own RSI nutrition plan is something you can control. It is something you can do to help yourself.

Why You Need More Nutrients Than Others Do

When you have RSI, the usual amount of nutrients needed to keep a healthy body in good working order is no longer sufficient. Your daily nutritional intake is quickly used up combating shock, tissue damage, and other issues facing your injured body. This leaves you with a system that is weakened and vulnerable. Simply put, your body is working overtime rerouting needed resources to its injured areas. So you have to take extra care to provide your system with the food it needs to heal.

Professional athletes understand these facts and regularly take vitamins and other nutritional supplements to boost their energy and help repair the damage that happens all too often when playing professional sports. In addition, they eat foods their bodies can absorb and burn efficiently. For example, before a marathon, runners load up on complex carbohydrates like pasta, peas, grain, and corn. These foods are perfect for long-distance runners as they yield energy for exercise over a prolonged period of time while keeping the blood sugar at a stable rate. They also provide a greater supply of muscle glycogen, your body's fuel, than do simple carbohydrates or sugars.

If you were a famous baseball player, earning millions of dollars a year, the doctors would have ice packs on your pitching arm before, during, and after the game. They would provide massage therapy, special nutritional supplements, and a prescribed diet to keep you fit. They would recognize your body as an important tool in your physical and mental work. So why don't we accord ourselves the same respect? *The New York Times* (August 1996) proclaimed musicians as the "fine motor athletes of today." But you don't have to be famous or even play the violin to take care of yourself. The RSI epidemic is affecting all of us in the work force, regardless of fame or paycheck. Let's make sure we are giving our bodies all the nutritional help we can.

Again, as an RSI sufferer, you might find it useful to start thinking of yourself in the same way an athlete does. Over the years, you have moved in the same way, accumulating trauma to the same muscles, tendons, and ligaments until it blossomed into some form of RSI. You have the same amount of pressure and emotional investment in your level of productivity and quality of performance as a professional athlete and the RSI is now threatening your work. To reach your optimal level of health and performance you should have a nutrition plan that is designed especially for you, the RSI worker. A healthy, low-fat, low-cholesterol diet is a good nutritional starting place.

Every choice you make at the table impacts upon your ability to resist illness, to maintain a high energy level, and to heal. The food you eat affects your appearance, your stamina, and your overall feeling of well-being. While there is no single vitamin or pill that will cure your RSI, there are nutrition plans that can facilitate your healing and others that will retard it.

When your body is injured, it needs different nutrition—not necessarily more calories—in order to heal itself. RSI sufferers are more vulnerable to overeating than other people. When you are in chronic pain from RSI, weight gains of anywhere from twenty to forty pounds are not unusual. These extra pounds stay on because patients convince themselves that eating and total rest make them feel better. And, in a way, food does make you feel better. Junk food certainly provides emotional comfort with its connotation of deserved self-indulgence. This often offers temporary relief from the depression so commonly accompanying RSI. Other foods also increase the amount of serotonin, the natural antidepressant in the brain. Serotonin makes endorphins, pain-fighting, feel-good hormones, and you really may feel less pain when your mouth is full. But after the initial feeling of relief, the effect reverses itself and you will experience more pain.

If you're engaged in an ongoing battle with the refrigerator, you may wonder if you have the emotional and mental stamina to lose weight and manage your RSI pain at the same time. Here are two good reasons to try:

• Every extra pound you put on strains the muscles that have been injured and weakened through disuse.

• Overeating actually sabotages your major goal of getting better. It is an actual assault on your body.

The Nine Goals of the RSI Diet

1. Have six small meals throughout the day and two snacks.
2. Eat moderate-sized portions at each meal.
3. Load up on vegetables and proteins.
4. Avoid saturated fats and cholesterol.
5. Eat as much fish as you can.
6. Cut back on simple carbohydrates.
7. Avoid caffeine, colas, refined sugars, and salt.
8. Cut out cigarettes and alcohol.
9. Drink eight glasses (2 liters) of water per day.

Each body has different needs, different nutritional requirements. Sit down with your doctor. Tell him you want to optimize your body's ability to heal itself. See if he has any specific nutritional supplements for you. Ask for a mineral/vitamin workup—it is a simple blood test that could hold the key to your well-being. Everyone responds to supplements differently. If you are having a side effect after adding a supplement to your regimen, call your doctor immediately. The body is an extremely complex machine that, like a fine car, needs constant retuning and adjusting. Be patient and you will arrive at the nutritional formula that is best for you and your RSI.

Below are nine easy goals to slowly integrate into your daily routine. You should consider each of equal importance.

Goal 1: *Have six small meals throughout the day and two snacks.*

Six small meals: You need more energy when you are injured. Your body uses more fuel to heal itself; you tire easily and need constant "refills." That's why eating six small meals spread throughout a day provides more benefits to healing your RSI than three big repasts.

Goal 2: *Eat moderate-sized portions at each meal.*

You need 1,200 to 2,000 calories per day—depending on your individual size, sex, and activity level. Check with your physician for the appropriate daily calorie intake *for you*, then pay attention to your calorie intake at each meal so that you don't go above your daily intake level.

The human body is built from the nutrients it gets from food: water, protein, fat, carbohydrates, vitamins, and minerals. About 60 percent of your weight is water, about 20 percent of your weight is fat, and about 20 percent is a combination of mostly protein plus carbohydrates, minerals, and vitamins. Your *nutritional status* is a term used to describe the state of your health as it relates to your diet. The amount you eat each day is measured in two distinctly different ways. For example, the recommended dietary allowance (RDA) is measured in micronutrients. Vitamins and minerals are in this group and are measured in anything from milligrams (1/1,000 of a gram) to micrograms (1/1,000,000 of a gram). RDAs vary among men and women of different ages. For example, because women of childbearing age lose iron when they menstruate, their RDA for iron (15 mg) is higher than that for the average male (10 mg).

The second way food is measured is in macronutrients (*macro* meaning big.) Your daily requirements for macronutrients generally exceed one gram. For example, the RDA for protein is set in terms of grams of protein per kilogram (2.2 pounds) of body weight. Because the average man weighs more than the average woman, his RDA for protein is higher than hers. The RDA for protein for the average male, age twenty-five to fifty, is 63 grams; for a woman, it's 50 grams. Macronutrients measure proteins, fats and oils, carbohydrates, and water. RDA minimal daily requirements are often incorrect since these standards badly need updating. It is important that you always check with a nutritionist and/or your physician before beginning any vitamin or mineral regimen.

Some nutritionists believe that RDAs are safe and effective and generous enough to prevent deficiencies but not so high that they will trigger side effects. Others believe that they are too low for optimal health. If you are serious about taking vitamins and minerals, you should sit down with a certified nutritionist and discuss what your treatment should be.

Goal 3: *Load up on vegetables and proteins.*

Protein makes up three-quarters of our body tissue and one-fifth of our weight. That's quite a lot of mass to support, especially since our bodies cannot store proteins, necessitating a new supply each day. If your diet does not contain sufficient amounts of proteins, you start to digest the proteins in your body, including the proteins in your muscles. RSI raises your protein requirements. An injured body releases above-normal amounts of protein-destroying hormones. With the extra protein in your RSI diet, you can protect existing tissues and generate new muscle tissue.

On average, protein should make up about 12 to 15 percent of your daily calories. There are many vegetable and nonmeat sources of protein so don't think you have to start a diet of pure meat. Because red meat is naturally high in saturated fats, keep your red-meat intake to under seven ounces per week. Lentils, chickpeas, beans and rice (together a complex protein that the body uses efficiently), tofu, cheese (choose the low-fat kind such as yogurt cheese), eggs, roasted peanuts, low or nonfat yogurt are a few nonmeat substitutes with high protein content.

Goal 4: *Avoid saturated fats and cholesterol.*

Our bodies convert the calories in dietary fat to body fat more efficiently than they convert the calories in carbohydrates and proteins. In other words, fats are more fattening. You need 67 grams or less, and no more than 30 percent of daily calories from fat. Each gram contains nine calories, more than twice the energy of carbohydrates or proteins. *Just stay away from saturated fat.*

All fats are a combination of **saturated** fats and unsaturated fats **(polyunsaturated and monounsaturated)**. Saturated fats are easy to

---

HERE ARE A FEW WAYS TO HELP YOU KEEP THE FAT OFF

- **Ask your butcher to trim the fat** from all your meats and poultry.
- **Reduce or eliminate your whole-milk products.** There are now nonfat substitutes for most whole-milk products that have enriched calcium and vitamin D and taste good.
- **Use olive or canola oils for cooking and salads.** These are low-cholesterol, low-saturated-fat oils.
- **If you like snacks, reach for an apple or other fruit.**
- **Instead of junk food,** try pretzels or unbuttered popcorn. Both are low fat and low cholesterol. More importantly, when you first open that bag of snacks, put handfuls of pretzels or popcorn into several smaller bags. Now you know what a serving size is. This prevents that hand of yours from wandering into the main bag without your even knowing it!

---

recognize—they are hard at room temperature. Remove the saturated fats from your diet; they are the BAD FATS. These troublemakers have been linked to high blood cholesterol. They also add unwanted extra weight the quickest. With RSI, the less saturated fat you ingest, the quicker your body will heal itself.

It is easy to say you will cut out the bad fats in your diet. But the next moment you may find yourself munching on a chocolate bar or reaching for that delectable french fry. In reality, it is quite difficult to wean yourself away from your entrenched eating habits.

Here's a quick list of all-too-familiar foods that are high in saturated fats: butter, cakes and pastries, cookies, fried foods, potato chips, pork rinds, chopped chicken liver, sour cream, cream cheese, cheese, coconut oil, meat with lots of fat, duck, processed meats, and ice cream.

Ideally, we should avoid all saturated fat and include in our diet only monounsaturated and polyunsaturated fats. But every naturally fat-rich food contains a mixture of all three fats. Your strategy should be to try to balance the three. Remember: *Your total intake of food should contain no more than 30 percent of your daily calories from fat.* That 30 percent should have as little saturated fat as possible. The average American eats a diet with a polyunsaturated-to-saturated fats ratio of approximately one to seven. With RSI, we are aiming to change that ratio to one to one.

One of the most motivating factors for maintaining a low-fat diet is the high correlation scientifically proven between a high-fat diet and breast cancer, an imbalance of female sex hormones, and cancers of the reproductive systems. A high-fat diet also heightens the risk of heart disease and stroke.

Cholesterol is a waxy substance essential to our good health that plays an important role in protecting and generating cells, fatty tissues, organs, and glands. It protects the integrity of cell membranes, helps enable nerve cells to send messages back and forth to the brain, is a base on which you build steroid hormones such as estrogen and testosterone, and helps your gallbladder to absorb fats and fat-soluble nutrients such as vitamins A, D, E, and K.

But our predicament is that our bodies already produce sufficient amounts of cholesterol. *We don't need any additional cholesterol in our diets.* Too much cholesterol drains your body's strength and thus weakens its ability to heal. So keep the cholesterol to a minimum. You need 300 milligrams or less a day of cholesterol. A low-cholesterol reading (ask your physician what your cholesterol is and if it needs to be lower) will keep your whole system strong.

Losing weight will make you feel better and help reduce your pain. Carrying extra weight puts more strain on your system with the higher cholesterol and extra fat levels and will slow down your RSI recovery. But when we are in pain and have decreased mobility from RSI, most of us feel that adding one more restriction, such as an unfamiliar diet, is just too much. Pain is overwhelming at times. But remember your goal: You want to feel better. You want to be pain free and move easily. If you start walking and make the few changes in your portion size, in the fat and carbohydrate content of each meal, the weight will come off more easily than you expect and the rewards will be great.

Goal 5: Eat as much fish as you can.

Omega-3s are heart-friendly unsaturated fatty acids found in their greatest concentration in high-fat fish from cold waters such as salmon or mackerel. Studies so far indicate that omega-3s play an important role in keeping blood platelets from sticking, reducing the likelihood of blood clots that can lead to heart attacks. Many studies on joint-impacting diseases like arthritis suggest avoiding dairy products and red meats. Instead, it is recommended that patients suffering from these diseases substitute fish and vegetables. The fats, proteins, and other nutrients found in fish are easily burned in the body. Many of my patients who have followed these recommendations swear that their energy level heightened and depression lifted.

The fatty acids in omega-3s also help block inflammation. Supplements of omega-3 fatty acids have been shown to help those with rheumatoid arthritis. A recent study shows that patients taking 2.6 grams of omega-3 fatty acids showed significant improvement in their assessment of pain. The group taking omega-3 supplements was also able to lower its other anti-inflammatory medication. Depending on where your RSI is concentrated and its symptoms, this might be a viable therapy to discuss with your physician.

Fish rich in omega-3s are striped sea bass, sardines in fish oil, swordfish, lake trout, albacore tuna, and halibut. Fish and crustaceans (shellfish) in general are good for you, so if you happen to dislike all of the above, eat any kind of fish you want. Just eat fish. Broiled and baked fish are naturally low in calories, but make sure you analyze the fat content of any added sauces or stuffing. (No guidelines have been established as to how much omega-3s you need daily. At this point in time, no one has reported having too much. So enjoy!)

Packaged salsa or chutneys offer a good low-fat nutritious way to spice up broiled fish or steamed veggies. Using spices and fresh herbs other than salt opens up a whole new way of eating that is nutritious, interesting, and as satisfying as the fat-laden habits of old.

There has been some concern lately about the methylmercury level in seafood. The FDA suggests that if you vary the kinds of fish you eat and don't go on any fad diets, mercury levels should pose no problem to the average individual. Fish is so high in beneficial nutrients that the FDA endorses its consumption. However, if you are pregnant or intend to have children, the FDA suggests you avoid shark and swordfish as they could contain harmful levels of mercury. The FDA also recommends you limit your overall fish intake to seven ounces per week. To check on any recent developments concerning the environment and its effect on your food, call the FDA hotline: 1-800-332-4010.

Goal 6: *Cut back on simple carbohydrates.*

Carbohydrates also provide energy to the body. There are two kinds of carbohydrates: simple carbohydrates or sugars (you'll find these in lactose from milk, glucose and fructose from fruit, and sucrose from cane and beet sugar) and complex carbohydrates or starches (found in cereal, bread, rice, pasta, beans, and corn). Both types are converted to glucose, the main fuel for our bodies, but starches are healthier because, unlike the empty calories of sugars, they are usually accompanied by other nutrients. You need 290 grams; 55 to 60 percent of daily calories should come from carbohydrates with no more than 15 percent from sugars. But carbohydrates can also foster mood swings, so be moderate with your intake of these as well.

Simple carbohydrates are sugar filled and energy draining. They include cakes, candies, cookies, corn syrup, dried fruits, fresh fruits, honey, jam, jellies, molasses, soda, maple sugar, and table sugar. Fresh fruits are good for you if, like everything else, they are eaten in moderation.

It's easy to confuse simple and complex carbohydrate-rich foods. Complex carbohydrates are rich in nutrients and essential to good health. *Complex carbohydrates* are the "good" carbohydrates. They include beans, breads, carrots, corn, crackers, nuts, parsnips, pasta, peas, potatoes, sweet potatoes, and winter squash.

Goal 7: *Avoid caffeine, colas, refined sugars, and salt.*

The caffeine you find in coffee, chocolate, black tea, and cola triggers muscle spasms. You don't want that! It will just add to your pain. Try weaning yourself from these stimulants. You'll probably find that your energy will improve. You'll find that you don't "crash" as much, your mood swings will lessen, and your natural energy has a better chance of taking over.

An integral part of RSI is stress. Your goal is to find all that helps your muscles and tendons relax. Exercise, plenty of sleep, the right nutrition, and a sense of well-being will give you plenty of energy. You don't need this other stuff.

Sodium helps to maintain the body's balance of fluids and is also essential to good health. However, sodium often triggers water retention, which can aggravate your RSI symptoms putting pressure on those irritated tendons and injured tissues. So if you are prone to retaining

TRY HONEY AS A SUGAR SUBSTITUTE

If you have a sweet tooth, try honey rather than white or brown sugar. Honey, in its natural state, is nutritionally similar to white sugar (sucrose). However, it is also one of the sweetest natural energy sources found in nature. The advantage of honey, when compared to white refined sugar, is that it does not rob the body of vitamins in order to process it. This means your body works less and can use these honey supplies for energy. It also means you have more vitamins to use for more important healing processes. But here again moderation is the key.

Honey is 63 to 80 percent natural sugar, levulose, dextrose, and some sucrose, which are easily absorbed by the body with very little digestion needed to turn the sugars into glucose. One tablespoon of honey will supply 3.6 percent RDA calories, 5.5 percent carbohydrates, 1.8 percent iron, and significant amounts of B vitamins, amino acids, and enzymes if it is not pasteurized. You should store honey in a dry place as it readily absorbs moisture and will start to ferment. So if your sweet tooth acts up, reach first for naturally-occurring sugars in vitamin-packed fresh fruits. If you still need a kick, put a half teaspoon of honey in a cup of herbal tea.

---

water, cut out the salt. Some people are "salt sensitive" and it can lead to high blood pressure and an increased risk of stroke, heart disease, and kidney failure. Talk to your physician about this. A typical, non-salt-sensitive person needs no more than 2,200 milligrams (about 1½ teaspoons) a day. Read the labels on your packaged foods before buying.

Goal 8: *Cut out cigarettes and alcohol.*

Smoking is a habit to avoid as it will exacerbate all your RSI pain symptoms. The nicotine found in tobacco deprives your muscles of oxygen, which, you already know, can increase pain. Smoking makes exercising more difficult and adds to other health risks such as cancer and lung disease. Unfortunately, it is a difficult habit to break. Ask your physician for suggested pharmaceutical aids that will help you break your habit easily and fast. Getting rid of those cigarettes is just another way of investing in your new pain-free lifestyle.

Alcohol is a toxin and natural depressant. If you find yourself feeling apathetic, tired, or depressed, eliminate all alcohol from your diet. With

MORE SUGGESTIONS FOR YOU JUNK-FOOD ADDICTS

Junk food surrounds us. Entices us. Most of it is drenched in oil and fried or satu-rated with an overabundance of sugar. For a while this was only true in America. Now, french fries and Big Macs or their close relatives stretch their chemical-filled, greasy tentacles from Paris to Bombay. It seems much easier to eat a high-fat, high-cholesterol diet because the food is brightly packaged, easily noticeable, and accessible on every street corner. Grabbing that chocolate candy bar for a quick energy lift is too frequent in most of our busy routines. (A typical chocolate candy bar can consist of four bites equaling over 1,000 calories that are way over your 30 percent saturated fat content! That's almost your whole day's budget of calories right there.)

A special note about pizza: This is a food that's easy to handle, so many RSI sufferers grab a piece whenever they can. If you can't manage anything else, then eat a piece now and then so you get something in your body. However, be aware that one piece of pizza is high in cholesterol, salt content, and saturated fats and averages about one thousand calories.

It actually doesn't take much planning to eat well. Now that you know what all those nasty sugars and saturated fats do to you, let's see how we can easily avoid them. You do need to be motivated to make any kind of change. With my RSI patients, the strongest motivating factor is pain. So let's start stacking the nutritional odds in your favor and get you back to a pain-free life.

---

the depression that often accompanies RSI, alcohol is the last thing you need to add to your system. If you are looking to escape or relax, go for a walk, listen to some music, take a warm bath by candlelight, or spend an evening with friends.

Goal 9: *Drink eight glasses (2 liters) of water per day.*

Your body uses water to send electrical messages between cells so your muscles will move, your ears can hear, your brain can think, and so on. Water also regulates body temperature, lubricates your mov-ing parts, carries away wastes products, helps you digest your food, and dissolves nutrients to enable your body to use them efficiently. It also provides a medium in which biochemical reactions such as metab-olism can occur. Almost three-fourths of the water in your body is liquid between body cells or intracellular fluid. The rest is extracellular fluid. A healthy body has fluid balance—the right amount of fluid inside and outside each cell. If there is not enough water inside a cell, it will dry out and die. If there is too much water, if will burst. If you drink more water than you need, your body naturally adjusts and eliminates it through heavier urination. But if you don't get enough water, your body will let you know immediately. You will feel thirsty, your mouth may feel dry, and you might notice a reduction in urination. These are signals telling you your fluid balance is off and you need to drink more water.

If you are on a high-protein diet, as I suggest, you need extra water to eliminate the nitrogen compounds (ammonia) that are left over after the protein is synthesized. The liver, which converts the ammonia into urine that is then excreted, needs the extra water to do the extra work.

Who Benefits from Supplements?

You may benefit from supplements if you have RSI because you may not be eating enough and your system needs some "extras" to heal. You should definitely speak with your doctor about supplements if you notice that the pain and fatigue of RSI has caused your appetite to drop off. Other people who will benefit are premenopausal women, adult women (who may need calcium supplements), women who are pregnant or nursing, vegans (who may require B_{12}, a vitamin from meat, milk, and eggs that vegans don't get through their diet), and people with metabolic disorders (these disorders often change how you absorb vitamins and minerals). So check with your physician.

Vitamins

Vitamin C (ascorbic acid), as mentioned previously, protects against infection and speeds up the healing of wounds. It is essential for the development and maintenance of connective tissue. Vitamin C speeds up the production of new cells in wound healing, and, like vitamin E, is an antioxidant that keeps free radicals from connecting with other molecules to form damaging compounds that may attack your healthy tissues. Recent research demonstrates that one gram or more of vitamin C will enhance the healing of minor wounds, reduce inflammation, and improve recovery. Vitamin C also protects your immune system, helping you fight off infection, reduces the severity of allergic reactions, and plays an important role in the synthesis of hormones and other body chemicals.

When your body is under great stress, as in chronic pain, the body's blood levels of ascorbic acid often decrease. This is true for both men and women. Vitamin C helps boost alertness and increases concentration. A deficiency of vitamin C can, therefore, make you less attentive and dampen your mood. Vitamin C–rich foods are needed for the production of collagen, an intercellular cement that gives structure to muscles, blood vessels, bones, and cartilage. Vitamin C also aids in the body's absorption of iron.

Five servings of fresh fruits and vegetables a day will usually provide all the vitamin C you need daily. Research shows that when subjects got more, they excreted the excess in urine. When they received less, they stored the excess in their immune cells.

Vitamin C–rich foods

Cantaloupe • Broccoli and Cauliflower, cooked • Grapefruit and Cranberry juice • Parsley, raw, chopped • Kale, cooked • Tomatoes • Cabbage • Oranges and Orange juice • Brussels sprouts, cooked • Lemon juice • Mustard greens • Bananas • Red peppers • Kiwis

Vitamin A keeps your system working. It is a moisturizing nutrient. It helps to keep the linings of the colon, esophagus, gallbladder, kidneys, intestine, stomach, rectum, and urinary tract in shape. The kind of stress most RSI patients experience often affects their digestive tracts or stomach linings. Stress also can make you more vulnerable to urinary tract infections, kidney stones, and sore throats. Vitamin A encourages the secretion of digestive juices, which keeps your "plumbing" in tip-top shape.

Vitamin A–rich foods:

Broccoli, Kale, Spinach, Parsley • Milk • Turkey • Cantaloupe, Papayas, Peaches, Pumpkins, Apricots, Carrots • Beef liver • Tomato juice • Eggs • Yogurt

Vitamin D: There are two kinds of vitamin D: One is found in the food we eat and the other is manufactured by our bodies when they are exposed to sunlight. Vitamin D is stored by the body because it is fat soluble. As a result it can be quite toxic when taken in large doses for an extended period of time.

Vitamin D–rich foods:

Milk • Tuna, canned in oil • Calf's liver • Herring, Sardines, Salmon, and Cod liver oil • Cheese

Vitamin E: Research shows us that the most effective vitamin E has two forms of the vitamin: alpha- and gamma-tocopherol. Therefore, when you buy a vitamin E supplement in the store, make sure it has at least these two. Vitamin E keeps the immune system strong and may be an important aid in fighting cancer as well as guarding against free-radical damage. Vitamin E also helps maintain a healthy reproductive system, nerves, and muscles. Research studies in Israel have begun to show that taking only 600 mg of vitamin E produced a marked reduction of pain after only ten days. This study suggests that natural vitamin E is better absorbed by the body than the synthesized product. Everyone agrees that a safe level of vitamin E supplement daily is 400 to 800 international units (IU) levels. It is generally agreed that over 800 IU daily can become toxic.

Vitamin E–rich foods:

Asparagus • Avocados • Broccoli • Peanut butter • Almonds • Hazelnuts • Whole grain breads • Sunflower seeds • Wheat germ • Dried prunes

Selenium is essential to the health of the heart muscles and to aid vitamin E in the prevention of free-radical formation, which is a possible cause of cancer. The selenium content of food varies with the selenium content of the soil in which it is grown.

Selenium-rich foods:

Fish: cod, flounder, herring, tuna, oysters, mackerel, sole • Chicken, all cuts • Bread: rye, whole wheat, white • Molasses • Popcorn • Beef: all cuts • Ham • Milk, skim and whole • Mushrooms • Rice: brown and white • Walnuts • Lamb • Peanuts • Spaghetti • Pork • Cashews

Antioxidants and Free Radicals

Free radicals trigger or exacerbate damage to joints by indiscriminately destroying healthy tissue. They are formed by a combination of the body's own metabolism as well as exposure to pollutants, bacteria, radiation, and cancer-causing chemicals. Free-radical molecules latch on to other molecules robbing the healthy molecules of their electrons. This chain reaction creates more free radicals. If there are billions of these tiny "bites" over time, they can add up to major joint damage.

Free radicals are destructive to joint tissues attacking the synovial fluid (the "oil" enabling your joints to move with very little friction) causing a breakdown in the fluid's lubricating properties. They can also chip off pieces of collagen (the structural protein that holds us together) from the cartilage itself.

Antioxidants sop up and neutralize free radicals. Selenium and vitamins C and E are three antioxidants easily accessible through supplements and food. Another lesser known group of antioxidants are called bioflavonoids. These seem to protect cultured cartilage tissue from the onslaught of free radicals. Citrus fruits, green and black teas, green leafy vegetables, and onions are all rich sources of antioxidants. Cumin, found in curry, is a potent antioxidant whose anti-inflammatory effect matches phenylbutazone, a drug used to fight inflammation and pain. I suggest you discuss with your doctor the viability of using antioxidants to combat any symptoms of inflammation you have.

Other Nutritional Supplements to Discuss
with Your Doctor

In 1991, a report showed that 60 percent of all Washington state dietitians took multivitamins. The newer poll (1994) shows that 78 percent of Americans now believe that taking supplements will help maintain their health. The Kellogg Report estimates that dissemination of new nutritional information will save $20.5 billion in health-care costs. Obviously, we don't get all the nutrition we need from the food we eat. We now have proof that this former piece of information is pure myth. *Time* and *Newsweek* magazines ran articles emphasizing how the medical community is finally beginning to realize that nutrition and healing are inevitably and inextricably linked.

If you decide to take supplements, remember renewal is a slow and steady process. You have to be patient. You need to wait until the nutrients are absorbed and converted in your body's many systems for their real benefits to show.

Be aware that herbal and nutritional supplements can interact adversely with prescribed medication or negatively affect a condition or injury. An easy way to protect yourself, besides researching each supplement you take for yourself, is to consult your doctor. You may want to get his or her feedback and suggestions on the following supplements that have been helpful to some of my patients with RSI.

Pycnogenol is a popular anti-inflammatory used in France. It is made from pine bark. It tends to be rather expensive and there are few studies to back its pain-relieving claim. However, if you are searching for an alternative to other pain relievers for chronic RSI pain, you may want to discuss this supplement with your doctor.

Boron has some antioxidant and anti-inflammatory properties. It helps regulate certain hormones such as testosterone, estrogen, and calcitonin. A small study done by R. L. Travers and G. C. Rennie ("Clinical Trial—Boron and Arthritis" townsend lett.83 [1990]; 360) indicates that boron can cause significant improvement for those with osteoarthritis. It seems that the tissues in hip joints have a dense concentration of boron. Accordingly, stress on these joints might benefit from supplementation. Again, ask your doctor if boron will help *your* RSI symptoms.

Magnesium is key in the development of the musculoskeletal system including bones, muscles, and other soft tissues. Surveys report that up to 30 percent of the adult population studied have low levels of magnesium. Therefore, you may benefit from a regular dose; discuss the possibility with your doctor.

Silicon has been recently recognized as performing an important role in strengthening connective collagen tissues and the mineralization of bone. There is not much research on silicon so I suggest you boost your intake through diet or take a low dosage of 5 to 10 mg per day. Silicon is found in sand (silicon dioxide) and eaten when it is inadvertently left on vegetables and fruit such as spinach, kale, and lettuce. Sand causes no known adverse effects.

Zinc: The majority of studies indicate significant benefits from taking zinc such as the reduction of joint pain and tenderness. Zinc is involved in cartilage metabolism and serves, with copper, as a vital component to help certain enzymes work properly. Talk to your doctor about the advisability of a zinc supplement in your case.

Fish-oil supplements (omega-3s): There have been many studies done regarding fish-oil supplements and inflammation, joint tenderness, and stiffness. The effects are moderate but significant. This research involved studies of patients with rheumatoid arthritis. Taking ten to fifteen fish-oil capsules daily decreased participants' joint tenderness, reduced stiffness in the morning, and eventually allowed a diminished reliance on anti-inflammatory drugs and pain medications. RSI is not arthritis but some of the triggers for swelling, inflammation, joint tenderness, and stiffness are similar. Accordingly, omega-3s may help your condition. Fish-oil supplements (polyunsaturated fats) are also needed to make hormonelike substances called *prostaglandins*. The good type of prostaglandens help the immune system do its job fending off disease, fighting infection, and reducing inflammation.

Cayenne (capsicum): A special word about cayenne. Many over-the-counter creams and gels are popping up with capsicum as the main ingredient. Recently, studies have shown that, when used externally, creams containing capsicum relieve pain associated with osteoarthritis (of the hands), reflex sympathetic dystrophy (RSD), and pain associated with RSI (of the hands and shoulders).

Little research has been done in pain management directly related to RSI. Thus, we often have to look at similar injuries or conditions, like arthritis, to judge the beneficial effects of new treatments. In 1992, the *Journal of Rheumatology* reported that pain and tenderness were reduced by about 40 percent for those with painful arthritis of the hands who used cayenne supplement versus those not treated.

Cayenne is a beneficial and powerful botanical and should be treated with respect, whether taken in cream form or capsule. Because capsicum cream can burn, take care when applying it and wash your hands afterward to avoid getting it in your eyes or other sensitive areas such as open cuts, lesions, or sores. Before using these creams, make a test area in the crook of your elbow or some other sensitive spot since some people react to cayenne with a violent rash. If this occurs, you should stop using it immediately. Otherwise, use according to directions and it may help with your pain.

Boswellin cream is a topical cream sold in health-food stores that has proven effective for some who are combating RSI pain. It is an extract from *Boswellia serrata* gum resin containing a minimum 65 percent boswellic acid as the active principle. The boswellia tree grows wild on dry hills throughout most of India. From this tree comes a nonsteroidal compound that has been found effective in treating various forms of inflammation of the joints, without side effects. There was also a study with a mixed group of subjects (five to seventy-five years old), reporting a 97 percent increase of movement after supplementing the participants' diet with boswellic acids. In these groups, boswellic acids reduced discomfort and morning stiffness, and improved grip strength and physical performance. The topical cream soothed pain and inflammation. The RSI patients of mine who have tried this topical cream report a variety of results, from "it took the pain away for hours" to "it dulled my pain and reduced inflammation" to "it didn't work for me." More studies obviously need to be done but boswellin cream is benign enough for you to try if you want another alternative treatment for reducing pain and inflammation.

Now you know what you should eat. I have introduced you to various motivating factors to eat "right" and to some of the supplements that can help your RSI symptoms. Next, let's look at the role nutrition plays in mental health.

Mental Health, RSI, and Nutrition

One of the nasty side effects of RSI is depression. When depression hits, all motivation evaporates. But as you recognize what is happening to you, you can take the first step to change your life. Recognize that much of what you are feeling may be due to a *chemical depression*. In other words, your feelings are real but perhaps the triggers to those feelings are due to a chemical imbalance rather than a pure emotional reaction. When you change your intake of nutrition, you have a good chance of ridding yourself of these awful feelings. *Foods can affect your mood.*

Depression manifests itself differently in each person but whatever form it takes, it should be treated with attention. Caffeine, chocolate, and sweetened foods, besides contributing to muscle spasms, trigger a rapid rise in blood sugar. The familiar "crash" that follows a few hours later fuels wide mood swings. Other prompts can be unknown food allergens such as wheat and dairy, or chemicals in those artificial colorings and preservatives. Although these are unlikely to trigger a clinical depression, they can maintain low-grade depression or magnify an existing unbalance.

Depressed people are often "carbohydrate cravers." If you suspect this describes you, try eating fewer simple carbohydrates and more vegetables and protein. Vitamin deficiency can also mimic depression. Make sure your doctor checks your mineral and vitamin levels, especially B_3 and B_{12}. Vitamin B complex is critical to mental health as are vitamin C and essential minerals like calcium, magnesium, and potassium.

While carbohydrates tend to make the blood sugar level rise and fall, protein helps to rebalance it. This makes for a more stable psyche. Talk to your nutritionist about the amount and kinds of protein you eat.

An herb that has been showing success lately in helping to lift depression while you are rebalancing your system with vitamins and your altered nutritional intake is Saint-John's-wort. This herb has a long tradition of use in Europe as an antidepressant; it acts as an inhibitor of a brain enzyme, monoamine oxidase (MAO), similar to many antidepressant medications. Raising the level of these enzymes for a short while appears to lift moods. Balancing them over the long run appears to help people to heal from depression.

The Importance of Attractive Food

Research clearly shows us that when we find our food attractive, no matter what the specific food or portion size, we are more satisfied. Since RSI symptoms can cause feelings of apathy and fatigue, it is often hard to feel any enthusiasm about fixing an appealing meal because of malaise and lack of mobility. You may find that you often tend to snack because you simply don't have the energy or interest to fix attractive food. But when you eat regular meals and eat well, many of these feelings will recede and this contributes to your overall return to health.

We've looked at how different foods can boost your spirits; sometimes the way you present and prepare your meals can have an uplifting effect as well. Here are some tips on how to make your food more enticing and satisfying with a limited amount of effort.

• Keep a bunch of fresh parsley in a glass of water with a plastic bag over it in the refrigerator. Parsley is great for keeping the kidneys and bladder clear as well as acting as a breath freshener. It is also loaded with calcium and potassium. Parsley is used by many of the great chefs to dress up plain-looking food. Try it in your own kitchen.

• We've come a long way from the awful-looking plastic tableware of the '60s and '70s. There are inexpensive, light, attractive dishes, glassware, and silverware that you can buy to perk up your everyday meals. (See Catalogs in the appendices.)

• Pay attention to color as well as nutrition. Store-bought salsas and chutneys make steamed vegetables into an exciting dish.

• Plan your food preparation time so that you're not exhausted and in pain by the time the food is ready. This means lots of rest breaks and maybe preparing part of the meal a day ahead as well as keeping extra sauces and chopped vegetables in the freezer.

• Share your food with someone. Food is innately more enjoyable when shared with a friend. Try not to eat alone. You'll eat slower, digest better, and have more fun.

Now let's find out about other ways to balance, stretch, limber, and relax our RSI systems. The next chapter is all about how to adapt traditional yoga positions to RSI needs and limitations. Yoga helps us take care of many of the emotional, spiritual, as well as physical challenges that RSI poses every day.

7. Step Six: Practice Safe and Easy Yoga for RSI

Yoga is more than five thousand years old and a recent poll tells us that it is enjoying huge popularity in this country with over six million Americans practicing yoga on a regular basis. Originally designed in India as a means to strengthen the body for long periods of meditation, calming both the mind and nervous system, yoga is now used as exercise worldwide benefiting the general health of all ages. I find many of my patients turning from aerobics to yoga as they complain that aerobic classes are too hard on their knees and lower back. Yoga is gentler on the joints and increases strength, flexibility, and muscle tone as well as calming the spirit. It is perfectly suited for RSI sufferers or those at risk for RSI.

The reason many of my patients were injured with RSI was due to overwhelmingly fast-paced, continuous activity. I began prescribing yoga in order to teach them how to slow down. As I became familiar with yoga's benefits, I realized that it helped to retrain my patients to move efficiently while relaxed. Most patients need to increase their awareness of their body's tension, pain, and stress and ease up when they realize their body is experiencing these negative sensations. They need to learn how to nurture their bodies' energy and provide their muscles with sufficient amounts of oxygen to prevent lactic acid buildup. The more conscious of themselves they become, the easier it is for my patients to heal and prevent reinjury. I have seen this time and again. Yoga provides the RSI sufferer with the perfect means to do all this and more.

This chapter's goals may take some perseverance but will take you further on your path toward recovery. Your will need to look for a yoga class and instructor that fits your needs and to discuss the various yoga asanas or positions you learn with your physical therapist. He/she may be able to adapt the positions to your present range of movement and weight-bearing limitations more easily than your yoga instructor. But ask both for help. Integrate these exercises into your morning and evening routines and then choose which ones work best for you. As with anything new, the only way you will know if yoga will help is to try it.

Practicing Adapted Yoga Poses for RSI

Yoga is uniquely noncompetitive. You don't have to keep up with anyone but yourself. This is particularly important to those with RSI since many of us are our own worst enemy pushing ourselves and our bodies beyond their limits.

Yoga practice is comprised of a series of strengthening and stretching poses performed sitting, standing, or lying down. These poses can be adapted to any skill level and provide benefits when practiced even for a short period each day. The poses included in this book are just a few that I offer with RSI's special requirements in mind. If you practice them regularly they should add energy, decrease your pain, strengthen and stretch your muscles, and help you to relax. I suggest you set aside fifteen minutes when you first awaken in the morning and then at night, before you go to sleep. The restorative yoga practice recommended here places minimal metabolic demands on you unlike most other kinds of exercise. Its soothing, stretching benefits will help you recover from the emotional drain and fatigue imposed by RSI. It might even inspire you to explore the practice of yoga more fully as you continue to heal and grow.

HOW DOES YOGA WORK?

With its emphasis on deep breathing and meditation, yoga helps you become aware of your mind and body connection, which can offer you potential relief of pain. Yoga focuses on body awareness, gently allowing you to find your body's center and align yourself to it, and gradually increases your feelings of being grounded and in control during your RSI recovery and beyond. The stretches and relaxations involved in practicing the breathing techniques and yoga asanas (positions) help tone, strengthen, and heighten your flexibility.

Many of my patients report that they start yoga for RSI relief but continue for pure enjoyment.

We know from research that thought and emotions directly influence physiological responses, including muscle tension, blood flow, and levels of certain calming brain chemicals. All of these dynamics play important roles in the production and suppression of pain. The practice of yoga helps you gain greater control over many of these processes by making you more aware of your mind's and body's functions and working to slow and calm them. Psychological factors also indirectly influence pain by affecting the way you cope with it. Although the physical cause of pain may be identical within a group of individuals, the perception of pain and coping responses can be dramatically different. One man's ache is another man's nightmare. Yoga can give you a sense of control over your RSI pain by teaching you how to *let go* of it and concentrate on greater relaxation. As you learn this subtle skill, it enhances all of your emotional and physical abilities through RSI recovery and beyond.

Quite simply, the centuries-old practice of yoga happens to create an environment that encourages you to recover from RSI not only physically, but mentally and spiritually as well.

Finding the Yoga Teacher and Class for You

Finding the right yoga teacher is paramount. You may have no trouble at all. But you may have to try one or two instructors before you discover someone who is trained and willing to take the time to adapt the asanas to your injuries and limitations. Always observe a class before you decide to join. This is a common practice for first-time participants in a yoga class, so no one will think your request to do so is unusual.

Your attitude. Try to be relaxed, explicit, and direct about your needs when talking to yoga instructors. Especially if yoga is new to you, don't expect to feel comfortable with the discipline right away. It may take time but you should feel comfortable asking questions from the start. It is of paramount importance to explain to the instructor about any health limitation you have. If he or she is not willing to listen and respond to your satisfaction, keep looking for a class you can attend and for the information you need. Certain positions and exercises are not recommended for those with RSI and others are emphasized for different medical conditions. Your instructor should guide you through the poses so you don't extend yourself beyond your limitations. If the instructor doesn't know what RSI is, explain in detail, offer written information, or find an instructor who is familiar with it. The more informed you and your instructor are, the better the class will be.

The instructor's attitude. Determine if:

- The instructor seems comfortable discussing your needs.
- The instructor seems to understand what you are talking about, and if he or she doesn't, does he or she ask questions?
- Is he or she willing to create adaptations of the poses with you?
- Does this class have an environment in which you can ask questions and learn?

Ask yourself if you understand what the instructor is saying. If you don't understand, this is the wrong class for you. Each class will be a little different, so don't hesitate to search for a class in which you feel at ease with the pace and the instructor.

Since yoga is primarily focused on practicing poses and breathing technique rather than talking, it is important that you feel safe and confident to express yourself. If a position hurts you or is uncomfortable, you must tell your instructor immediately. He or she should then adjust the exercise to fit you or should help you move to fit the exercise safely. If this does not happen, find another class.

Other elements to notice while observing a yoga class you are considering joining:

• *Is the space warm enough for you?* As you know, many with RSI have severe cold sensitivity. In some yoga exercises, the body temperature drops naturally. Does the teacher provide blankets or remind you to bring a towel for warmth? You should get in the habit of having a covering handy to keep you at a comfortable temperature.

• *Does the class begin and end with breathing exercises?* This practice is particularly beneficial to those with RSI as it centers awareness and relaxes and warms the muscles before any stretching begins. This is not imperative but would be good to keep in mind. If the instructor does not start and finish with breathing exercises, you may want to arrive early and stay a little late to do them on your own.

• *What happens if you don't feel good after yoga or don't feel as if you are progressing?* Talk to your instructor and your physician. Your physical therapist might shed some light on your dilemma also. Your yoga class may be progressing too slowly or too quickly for your needs. Even if you *like* your yoga teacher, he or she may ultimately not be right for you. There are many yoga centers around the country that have lists of qualified yoga instructors. Look for the yoga class that emphasizes breathing techniques and seems more gentle than rigorous. You need the yoga class that is slow and steady and provides students with a lot of attention. Many times, the yoga teacher who doesn't fit your needs may know of a class and instructor who will. So ask.

Everyone has his own pace and perhaps you need more emphasis in an area that the rest of the class ignores. One of my patients was very adept at adapting yoga positions to her RSI. After two years in a restorative yoga class, she felt ready to join a "regular" yoga group. The teacher of the regular yoga class was so impressed with her ability to adapt that he ignored her! She learned nothing and felt she might as well be practicing yoga at home. After discussing this with her instructor, he explained that the class was too large for much individual attention and suggested another class, which turned out to be much better suited to her needs. So make the effort to find the best class for you. The initial time it takes will pay off later.

Yoga in a Seated Position

Susanne Chakan, a certified hatha yoga instructor in New York City, designed a course for newcomers to yoga with mobility impairments such as those caused by RSI. Her classes were small and all the initial positions were practiced seated on chairs. This was a perfect solution for those with RSI who couldn't and shouldn't be placing any weight on their arms, wrists, or shoulders, something that can easily happen when practicing poses while seated on the floor. Yoga floor poses can be adapted for RSI, but many of my patients found it easier in the beginning to sit on chairs. The benefits were the same and chairs that Susanne started with provided a concrete support reminding the student not to overreach his limited range of movement.

Susanne began every class with diaphragmatic breathing exercises (see chapter 4), which relaxed the students and put them more "in the moment," as the yogis like to say. She adapted arm stretches, spinal twists, and even balancing poses so her students were either standing or sitting for all of them. The pace of the class was especially unhurried, allowing each student to find the limit to his stretch and strength threshold before pain began. Each stretch was done slowly. The students were told to stop the exercise *before* the onset of pain. They were told to notice where each arm was placed so that later, in everyday movement, they wouldn't overreach and reinjure themselves.

There is usually quite a difference in flexibility and range of movement between the right and left arms in patients with bilateral injuries (both arms.) These yoga stretches for both sides of the body helped each student recognize his limitations for both right and left arms and work to gently improve mobility of each.

Throughout the class, Susanne strongly suggested relaxation exercises between positions (asanas). These were particularly important for RSI sufferers who usually compensate for the weaknesses on one side with the stronger limb on the other side. These enforced rest periods provide the whole body with a much needed time of relaxation. You may find that ever since you were injured, you tire more easily. Your yoga class should incorporate scheduled rest periods and you should include them in yoga practice at home as well. They should help to remind you that you need to slow down and rest more than usual. This is something that most of us find difficult to remember.

Some yoga poses are best done lying down on comfortable mats with pillows, rolled towels, or foam for support. Placing a rolled-up towel above your head while lying on your back is a physical reminder that will stop you from stretching your arms too far. Foam or rolled towels placed on your lap can support your arms when you are sitting, or place them under your arms when lying down similar to how you use pillows at home. Take as long as you need to determine the perfect combination of supports for you. Use this combination of supports in your office chair, on your couch or easy chair at home, and on your own bed when you find yourself awakened in the night wrestling with discomfort and insomnia. You may suddenly find yourself able to sleep through the night with minimal interruptions.

Any yoga class you take should also teach you breathing techniques that will help you return to sleep and other techniques that infuse the body with energy. You should feel better after the hour-long class. My patients who practice these adapted restorative poses at home find that they feel better. You will find some of the easier poses described at the end of this chapter.

There are many wonderful books on yoga on the market if you want to read about the subject on your own. Two of my favorites are *Relax and Renew: Restful Yoga for Stressful Times* by Judith Lasater, Ph.D., PT (Rodmell Press, 1995) and *Yoga Basics: The Essential Beginner's Guide to Yoga for a Lifetime of Health and Fitness* by Mara Carrico and the editors of *Yoga Journal* (Owl Books, Henry Holt and Company, 1997). I strongly recommend you try a class or two if you are suffering from RSI. Most of my patients report that their entire sense of well-being has improved since beginning yoga.

The Mind-Body Connection and Yoga

Yoga is an effective way of relaxing all that tension and restoring your health. It is that simple. Yoga, as Judith Lasater explains in her book, *Relax and Renew*, is "active relaxation." The body's capacity to heal itself is unlimited if we give it a chance. See if you can't add the yoga exercises in this chapter to your daily routine. You may be surprised how soon you find yourself looking forward to the relaxing benefits of regular practice. One of my patients summed up the benefits of yoga succinctly when she told me, "I just couldn't find a way to stop. I was constantly running from one thing to another. There seemed to be no time for me. Yoga gave me that time. Now I love doing my poses and breathing exercises. I feel as if I am actively healing when I do yoga. It is quite a gift."

Before and After Yoga

• **A word of caution.** Check with your physician before beginning yoga or any other kind of exercise. As benign as yoga can be, your particular injury may not be ready for certain poses. You need to recognize your limitations. Yoga is a good place to explore these limitations but be careful not to reinjure yourself. Be sure to keep a regular dialogue going with your doctor, physical therapist, and yoga instructor to accurately gage your progress and danger points. This way you can work yourself back to health with no setbacks.

• **What to wear when practicing yoga.** Wear loose, comfortable clothing that allows you to move freely and keeps you comfortably warm. In general, you can wear socks. If you are practicing in the office, loosen your tie or top button on your shirt or blouse and any buttons at your wrists. Loosen your belt and remove your shoes if it is appropriate. Remove your eyeglasses or contact lenses and wristwatch.

• **Should you eat before practice?** Wait at least two hours after eating before you begin practicing. Allowing time for digestion will enable you to breathe easier and feel more relaxed and comfortable.

• **Be careful about driving immediately after practicing relaxing poses.** You may be completely relaxed after practice so take some time to become fully alert before driving.

Yoga Poses for Prevention and RSI Recovery

Breathing for Energy and Relaxation

You already know how to breathe from your diaphragm (chapter 4). Now let's try an exercise that will energize you.

To start, find a comfortable position, lying on the floor or sitting in a chair. If you are sitting, make sure your head, neck, and spine are aligned and relaxed. In a sitting position, your feet should be flat on the floor and hands resting on your thighs.

• Close your eyes.

• Inhale deeply through your nose so your diaphragm expands. Exhale, pushing the air out from the diaphragm through your nose. Make this exhalation last as long as you can. Take a deep, natural breath and repeat the deep inhalation and long exhalation. Do this two or three times. It may make you a bit light-headed at first. If you find you are light-headed, decrease the breath repetitions to one or two until you are no longer light-headed. Don't increase the number of repetitions until your light-headedness disappears.

• When you have completed your breathing repetitions, you should be breathing naturally. Rub the palms of your hands together until you feel some heat being generated. Cup your palms over your eyes.

• Breathe in and, when you do, try and see if you can feel the heat from your hands being drawn in through your eyes. Then exhale.

• Open your eyes.

• With the tips of your fingers or thumbs, gently rub around the tops of your eyes and cheekbones.

• Put your hands down to rest and relax.

Try practicing this exercise before and after work. It should get your whole system pumping with energy.

Exercises for the Neck

Make sure you do these *slowly* while in a seated position on a chair. These exercises are great for those nasty muscle spasms and knots that build up in the neck from many kinds of RSI. The more relaxed and stretched your neck is, the more overall relief you will feel. The number of repetitions depends on the degree of involvement of your neck and shoulders. Begin with three repetitions. If three seem to exacerbate your condition, start with one and gradually increase to two. Concentrate on how you feel. You should only repeat the exercise if it triggers no pain. With time, you should be able to do three repetitions easily and more as you recover. But don't rush the process.

Side-to-side Stretch

• To begin, position your head so you are looking straight ahead, your head balancing comfortably between your shoulders.

• Take a deep breath.

• Exhale while dropping your *left* ear toward your *left* shoulder. Move slowly and don't extend beyond the point when you feel pain. Relax your shoulder. Feel the gentle pull on the right side of your neck.

• Remember to continue to breathe. With each exhalation, the neck muscles should relax a little more. Bring your head back to the center or neutral position on the next inhalation. This is a simple side-to-side stretch.

• Then repeat these movements on the left side. Before you start on the next stretch, take a few deep breaths with your head facing forward and notice the relaxation you feel.

Chin-to-Chest Stretch

• To begin, your head should be centered between your shoulders so you are looking straight ahead. Inhale deeply.

• On the exhalation, drop your head to your chest.

• Relax your shoulders. Feel the stretch in your upper back and neck.

• Keep on breathing. You should feel your muscles relax more and more on each exhalation. Your chin should move closer and closer to your chest.

• Don't push. After a few breath cycles, inhale as you lift your head back to the initial center position. Relax. Repeat three times.

Exercises for the Shoulders

Inhale and lift both shoulders up toward your ears. On the exhalation move them forward and down. Relax. Repeat twice slowly.

You can do the above exercise one shoulder at a time to heighten awareness of the strength and flexibility differences between each side.

RSI-Adapted Sun Salutation

This shoulder and arm/hand exercise is an adapted position (asana) that builds strength and flexibility. It is an adaptation of the *traditional sun salutation*. This series of asanas is usually performed standing. This is a seated version that will remove any stress or weight from the arms and shoulders.

• Sit comfortably on a chair with your feet resting flat on the floor and your hands on your thighs.
• Inhale as you extend your arms in front of you at chest level, palms down.
• Exhale as you move the arms out to each side of your chest or heart center, stretching your arms out through your fingertips. Your palms should be facedown, your shoulders should be relaxed.
• Inhale as you again extend your arms in front of you at chest level, palms down.
• Exhale as you bring your thumbs to your heart center with your fingertips touching. Your elbows are bent and out to the side.
• Repeat the first and second positions. Keep your shoulders down and stretch open your chest as you reach out.
• Keep your arms out to the side, palms down. As you inhale, turn your palms upward. Feel the weight of gravity as you balance imaginary balls on each palm. Exhale.
• As you inhale, lift your arms as high over your head as you can, and make a round, ball shape with your hands above your head as your

fingertips gently touch. Your palms face each other. Keep your arms raised as you exhale.

• Take a deep breath and, as you exhale, put your palms together in a prayerlike position. Then as if you are pulling the energy down in a vertical line in front of you through your heart center, bring your hands down, still in prayer position, to your chest level.

• Continue pulling your hands down past your heart center until your hands naturally separate. This point of separation is called your flexibility limit. As you separate your hands, you should feel a stretch in your wrists as you let the energy go.

• Breathe deeply resting your hands on your thighs or at your sides. Relax. Gradually work on this series until you can complete this whole exercise twice.

Torso and Spine Stretches

The Spine Stretch

• Sit in an armless chair with your hands resting on your thighs and your feet planted on the floor. Your feet should be approximately hip distance apart.

• As you inhale, feel your hips push toward the floor, while your spine lengthens, the top of your head stretching toward the sky.

• As you exhale, let your arms hang at your sides. Relax your shoulders and neck and torso.

The Adapted Half Twist

• Sit in an armless chair with your hands resting on your thighs and feet planted on the floor, hip distance apart.

• As you inhale, place your left arm on your right thigh or loosely hold the seat of the chair under your right leg. Take hold of the back of your chair with your right hand. Turn and look over your right shoulder.

• Still holding that position, exhale. You should feel this half twist in your torso and spine. Keep your shoulders relaxed and down. Inhale and exhale again staying in this position. Each time you exhale you should feel the stretch again as the muscles release.

• Release the twist by returning to the neutral position—your hands resting once again on your thighs as you face forward. Take a few deep breaths and relax.

• Then inhale and place your right arm on the left thigh or loosely hold the seat of the chair under your left leg. Take hold of the back of your chair with your left hand. Turn and look over your left shoulder.

• Still holding that position, exhale. Feel this half twist in your torso and spine. Keep your shoulders relaxed and down. The muscles will release more and more with each exhalation.

• If you experience any cramps, muscle spasms, or pain, relax your position and come back to center as you inhale. Then breathe deeply and relax. You might want to stand and walk around awhile to release the static muscles.

Neck, Shoulder, and Back Stretch/Release

• Seated in your favorite armless chair, bring your head to the center as you inhale.

• As you exhale, bend forward, letting your weight rest on your thighs and knees and let your arms hang on either side of your legs.

• Inhale and exhale in this position a few times. You should feel the tension release in your back, neck, and shoulders.

• As you inhale, straighten up slowly until you are sitting upright once more. Exhale and relax.

This is a great back stretch and muscle release. When you are tired in the office, try this wonderful revitalizing exercise.

Balance, Endurance, and Concentration

The Tree

The Tree asana helps us develop balance, concentration, and breathing strength. For those with RSI, it also helps develop muscle tone and dissipates spasms and pain by helping to integrate the mind and body through concentration and relaxed, focused breathing. Some prefer to perform this asana without socks. You decide which you like.

A *word of caution:* You may have difficulty lifting your arms over your head. Just lift your arms as far as you comfortably can. Don't overreach in any part of any exercise. And if you can't manage the "prayer" position, just put your hands together the most comfortable way you can. The exercise will benefit you regardless of how close to the ideal position you can get. As you improve and become strong and more flexible, you can do the exercise as it is ideally designed.

• Stand with your feet hip distance apart, your arms at your sides, facing forward, your shoulders and neck relaxed.

• Inhale and raise your arms in front of you at chest height so that your palms are facing each other.

• Exhale, placing your palms together and bringing your arms over your head as high as is comfortable for you. Press your shoulders down. Then pull your hands down in front of your face continuing down in a vertical line to your heart center, hands remaining in a prayer position.

• You are now standing with your hands in a prayerlike position at your heart center and your feet are slightly apart.

• As you inhale, place the bottom of your right foot on the inside of your left leg—in a trianglelike position.

• Exhale and find a point on which you can concentrate as you breathe. Breathe as you experience the perfect balance of your being. Feel your muscles relax as you embrace gravity and space. Hold this position for fifteen seconds at first, working up to longer periods of time as you become more adept.

• On the next inhalation, separate your hands, letting them fall to your sides and gently put your foot down on the floor.

• Gently shake out your arms and shoulders and relax.

• Repeat the Tree, balancing on the opposite leg.

• Gently shake out your arms and shoulders and relax.

To end your series of asanas, I suggest you lie down on your back on the floor (the corpse position) with your hands resting comfortably at your sides. Close your eyes and breathe deeply. As you inhale and exhale, experience the relaxation of your forehead, your cheeks, your mouth and tongue. Then move slowly down your body—through your neck, shoulders, arms, and hands, your stomach, hips, thighs, calves, and feet. Be aware of any muscle tension you may feel and allow the muscles to release. Give yourself a good five minutes to achieve this state of total relaxation. Enjoy the luxury of being at complete rest.

Yoga is one, time-tested way for you to increase your range of motion and release muscle spasms and cramps. Although the asanas are done slowly, most students feel invigorated and limber at the end of a yoga workout. If you practice the above exercises every morning for fifteen minutes, you will be surprised at your improved endurance, muscle tone, and flexibility. The next chapter provides you with some Western exercises that complement your yoga routine. These Western exercises will also improve your circulation, energy, and general feeling of well-being.

8. Step Seven:
Follow Your Personal
RSI Exercise Program

The best exercise program for RSI is one tailored to your individual needs. The most difficult aspect of exercising when you have RSI is learning to recognize when and where your pain begins and stopping at that moment. That's where the "love" comes into play. This is the time when you decide to care and love yourself and make yourself feel good. The old "punishment and pain equals gain" motto just doesn't work anymore. Ignoring the natural warning signals that your body so conscientiously sends out is not the way to take care of yourself. Too many of my patients pretend that the pain and stress they feel with RSI are just part of normal everyday wear and tear. Many think that a good night's rest is all they need to get well. Many of my patients tell me this repeatedly. They say it until they convince themselves in spite of the exact opposite advice I provide. However, you know better. You now understand exactly how RSI benignly accumulates and becomes a full-blown injury. Your heightened awareness of how you move at home and at work will help you prevent further injury as well as aid you in effectively dealing with your RSI symptoms.

Our Natural Warning Signals

The treadmill of daily life most of us are on is so fast paced that we tend not to listen to our body's built-in warning system. In addition, RSI's onset is so gradual that it can take years before our mind opens to receive our body's danger signs once again and becomes cognizant of the growing weakness, tears, and strains in our muscles, ligaments, and tendons.

Imagine a body without our gross warning signals, the ones that occur when we bend our arm back or overextend our knee. Arms and legs would swirl about, tearing ligaments and breaking bones right and left. The only reason we don't bend our elbows back at a right angle is because it hurts. Our body sends the signal to our brain to stop. Luckily, we learn fast. If we turn our head awkwardly and a pain shoots through our neck, we subconsciously adjust our movement and don't turn exactly that way again.

Your goals in this chapter are twofold: you must learn to relax while you move and you must start paying attention to sometimes subtle pain signals the moment they begin. Ultimately, you need to learn where your limits are during movement before the pain begins. Often, by the time RSI has set in, those movements that cause pain can be very slight and require a lot of attention to notice and then focus on the retraining of our muscles.

RSI and Sports Soft-Tissue Injuries

One of the main differences between RSI, incurred during an average working day, and a sports soft-tissue injury of a professional athlete is the conditions of the individuals *before* they are injured.

Athletes who exercise regularly are in good shape. Their muscles and other connective tissues are flexible, toned, and strong. Their circulation is usually good and their immune system hardy. They are taught to rest between repetitions, giving their soft connective tissues time to regenerate and relax. And because of all that, when they are injured, their bodies recuperate quickly and usually regain all of their functioning.

In contrast, typical RSI sufferers spend most of their time doing one kind of work in a fairly static position. Few of them *warm up* for work. Deadlines make their movements smaller and tighter. Their activities rarely vary, so besides not moving enough, or resting enough, they rarely give their muscles the chance to stretch and flex in broad or gross gestures. They move repetitively at a pace too fast for the bodies to recover and mend any tissue tears in between. They are often in such poor condition that when they become injured, their systems don't have the resources to fully recuperate. Their weak bodies break down. Their connective tissues are tight, scarred, and weakened, restricting movement and causing pain. Their cardiovascular systems are not the best, and probably their general circulation could be greatly improved. The daily habits of many RSI sufferers leave them highly prone to RSI. And they heal slowly because of their overall lack of fitness.

Therefore, when a fit, sports-oriented individual is injured, the physical therapist will probably put him or her on weight-bearing exercises fairly soon after the trauma. However, with most RSI patients, experienced health-care professionals discourage this kind of exercise until the whole system has been built back to a relatively strong fitness level with months of gentle stretching and strengthening exercises.

This kind of overall weakness I've just described is a big concern for most of my patients with RSI. Perhaps you face the same drained physical state. However, remember that the overwhelming weakness you feel is mainly a symptom of RSI that you can condition away. It stems from passages that have become blocked by tissue that is thick, swollen, and fibrous as well as from compressed nerves. The lactic acid buildup makes you feel heavy and fatigued.

I know it's difficult to be objective about your recovery when you start out in great pain, slightly depressed, and exhausted. But understanding is your key. Now that you know what's going on, you also know that you need to keep moving and stretching in order to regain your strength. You also need to give yourself enough total rest time for your newly stretched and exercised muscles to heal. You need all of the proper nutrition and movement to wash away that toxic waste buildup in your limbs and get your circulation going again. Then you need to sleep and recover so you can begin again. Get the picture?

A guidebook I once read on how to survive in the mountains mentioned that one's state of mind is as important as all the physical aspects of a process when you have great difficulties to overcome. Recovery from RSI also begins in the mind. Attitude is an extremely important aspect in determining how you feel as you recover and how long that recovery takes. Retrain your muscles to lift your arm, use a pen, pick up a fork, or turn a page. I have seen many do these things and you can, too. Each painstaking step can be made, but first you must commit yourself to the psychological and spiritual process of becoming well. Once you have taken that first, all-important step, you will benefit a great deal from yoga and the exercises outlined here.

Hand Budgets and Exercise

RSI imposes restrictions on movement that if not treated may cause longer-term problems such as muscle atrophy, aggravated arthritis, or bursitis. I hear my patients talking about the amount of movement they can make at work or at home without incurring pain or discomfort; I refer to this as their hand "budgets." My patients tend to rest. Rest is good, I tell them, but why not stretch or limber while you are resting? Moving in a *different* way can reduce your RSI symptoms more often than complete rest. It is very important to remember that exercising safely will prevent weakness and atrophy and speed healing. That's why walking is so good for you. It increases circulation and improves your strength as you relax. Walking is an easily *managed* exercise. You can avoid hitting the ground too hard thus softening the vibrations that are naturally aggravating to RSI. You can practice being "aware" of how you feel as you walk. You can gently give your body the tone and strength it needs to return to full health. But walking is not the only exercise you can manage in this way and not the only one beneficial to your recovery. Yoga is another, and in this chapter we'll cover still more ideas.

Anyone can follow an exercise program in therapy, but few RSI patients I've seen can move throughout their day with relaxation and awareness. It is time you learned to do just that so you can benefit from all the experts who are offering you therapies to help you heal now and far beyond the time you stop seeing them. Follow these exercises and you will be on the way to a more rapid recovery and a more complete understanding of your individual injury and its limitations. This understanding of your own condition will also help you to train yourself against reinjury as well.

Limbering

Limbering is a slow, deliberate, gentle stretching combined with diaphragmatic breathing (breathing so your belly expands and your chest remains relatively still as you inhale). As I've mentioned before, deep breathing greatly increases the power of these exercises. So take the time to check on your breathing regularly as you practice them. Limbering prepares your body for more extensive stretching and more vigorous exercise. Whether you are injured or not, I strongly suggest you begin any period of movement with limbering. It allows you to test your limits before you exercise and prepare your body for movement. You can use limbering to slowly build up and meet your exercise goals in a safe, low-risk manner. Enthusiasm is great but so is education. Be a smart athlete. Take the extra time to warm up.

First, Relax

I suggest that you begin limbering by lying comfortably on your back. If you are not comfortable flat on your back, try putting extra pillows under an arm or leg or as a support for your head and neck. Some of my patients use six pillows as different props to reach their comfort zone. It is best to work without shoes and to keep the room temperature a bit warmer than usual if you are cold sensitive. This should help prevent muscle cramps and allow you to move more easily. Your hands should lie loose at your sides. Take three slow diaphragmatic breaths. Notice where you are holding tension and relax those parts of your body with each exhalation. Concentrate on letting all of the tension you feel float away.

RELAXATION DOS AND DON'TS

Dos

Do wear loose-fitting clothing.
Do modify the movement if you feel any discomfort.
Do recognize the wonderful feeling as all the tension leaves your body.
Do relax your face, jaw, and tongue. They, too, are part of you.
Do enjoy yourself as you are contributing to your recovery.

Don'ts

Don't wear shoes.
Don't stop exercising unless you can't avoid creating pain.
Don't grind your teeth or groan.
Don't sigh or get mad if you can't complete an exercise.

General Pointers about Limbering and Stretching

• Never shake out your hands if they cramp or hurt. Gently massage them. Run them under warm water or slowly open and close a fist.

• Invest in an exercise mat if you are exercising at home. The surface you work on should be firm but comfortable. You should *not* work on a soft mattress that will stress your lower back and neck giving them too little support. A floor with no mat is usually too hard and uncomfortable.

• Keep a couple of towels rolled up near you while you stretch or limber. Depending on your range of mobility, it is often more comfortable to slip a towel roll under your arm when lying flat on the floor. Take time to experiment as to where you need the extra height or support. If you are having trouble with your neck, it often helps to put a small rolled towel underneath your neck so that your head is slightly supported and there is no pull on your upper vertebrae.

Your Home Treatment Program

Your physical therapist has, by now, provided you with special exercises that are tuned to your individual injuries. I suggest you use your new yoga exercises to relax in the morning followed by your special exercises and the stretching and limbering routines provided below. The whole routine offers you thirty to forty-five minutes of home care daily. I suggest that you try this routine in the morning and before bedtime. It will help you pace yourself, move with efficiency throughout your day, and sleep better.

Three Times Each Unless You Are in Pain

Here are limbering exercises that will help teach your muscles to move and release while relaxed. This should help stop any pain you feel and allow your muscles to relax further. As a result, these exercises will help you learn how *to feel your body as you move* and teach you to determine how much you can move before triggering pain. With most of these exercises, I suggest three repetitions. If an exercise causes any pain, reduce the repetitions to two, and when there is no more pain response at that level, increase the repetitions.

Limbering the Neck and Trapezius Muscles

- Lie flat on your back in a relaxed comfortable position.
- Take a deep diaphragmatic breath. As you exhale, turn your head to your right shoulder as far as you can without pain. Find the degree that is comfortable and hold your head in this position until just *before* the pain begins.
- Then inhale and bring your head back to center.
- As you exhale, turn your head to the opposite shoulder. Again, find the degree of "turn" that is right before the pain begins. Hold your head there for the count of three.
- Inhale and return to center. Take two deep breaths.
- Repeat this exercise three times.

This exercise is particularly good for relieving muscle spasms around the top cervicals of the neck.

Shoulder and Upper-Arm Stretch

- Lie flat on your back in a neutral relaxed position.
- Slide your arms out to as close to shoulder height on each side as is comfortable. Your palms should face up.
- As you inhale, touch your left shoulder with the fingertips of your right hand.
- As you exhale, return your arm to the floor.
- Take a deep breath and relax.
- Then inhale and repeat with the other hand.
- You may not be able to reach the shoulder. Don't worry. Just extend as far as you can without triggering pain.
- Repeat three times.
- Each time you return your arm to the floor, make sure your whole arm, shoulder, and torso relax.
- Give yourself time to breathe in between repetitions until you feel totally relaxed.
- Remember to alternate hands. Doing this exercise three times consecutively with one hand may be too much strain.

This exercise will help you become aware of the movement limits of your shoulders and upper arms during the day so that you are not constantly reinjuring yourself as you heal.

Shoulder Rotation Exercise

- Lie comfortably on your back with your arms stretched out at shoulder height on the floor.
- Bend your elbows so your fingertips point to the ceiling and your elbows are at right angles to the floor.
- Gently lower your forearms down to the floor, palms down. Feel your shoulders rolling forward as you lower your arms. If your elbows are sensitive, you may want to place a soft towel under each of them for comfort. Don't push yourself past your limit.
- Be aware and notice that each arm may have a different range of

movement. One arm may not reach the floor, the other may touch it comfortably. Stop the movement in either arm if you feel pain.

• After determining your range of motion for each arm, you can use pillows to stop your arm from lowering any further than is comfortable for you.

• As you inhale, rotate your forearms back up, returning your shoulders back to neutral position. You should feel your shoulder blades and rotator cuffs move comfortably. Exhale.

• Take a deep breath between movements and relax completely.

Note: If you hear joints "cracking" don't worry; this is just your muscles readjusting to unfamiliar movements.

• Lower your forearms above you so your arms and the backs of your hands touch the floor or come as close to the floor as is comfortable. Rotate your shoulders back with this movement. Again, don't push. Just go as far as is comfortable.

• This exercise may be too painful for those of you with thoracic outlet syndrome. As you recover, you may try this exercise once a week to see if your condition has improved and you can then add it to your routine.

• For others, repeat three times.

Shoulder and Biceps Stretch

• Lie flat on your back with your arms down at your sides, palms up.
• As you inhale, make a fist and bring your fists up to your shoulders (upper arms still resting on the floor).
• Tighten all your arm muscles and squeeze.
• Exhale and release.
• Relax and repeat three times.

The Full-Body Stretch

• Lie flat on your back with your arms down at your sides. Palms up.
• Relax and breathe. Feel your whole body relax and sink to the floor. Focus on any area where you are holding tension; breathe and relax.

• As you inhale, slowly lift one arm at a time over your head as far as it will go.

• If you feel pain before your hand reaches the floor above your head, put a rolled towel or pillow above your shoulder to remind you not to move past your pain trigger point. This support will also relieve the "weight stress" created by lowering your arm over your head.

• Exhale as you return the arm to your side. Repeat this exercise with the other arm.

• Notice how far each arm will go. Be gentle. Don't push. Just be aware. Make sure your shoulders and neck are completely relaxed between repetitions.

• Repeat three times.

The Shoulder Shrug

• Lie on your back with your arms at your sides, knees bent, and your feet flat on the floor.

• Relax and take two deep breaths.

• As you inhale, slide your shoulders up as close to your ears as you can.

• As you exhale, slide your shoulders down until they are relaxed.

• Repeat twice.

• Take a deep breath and exhale.

For all the exercises in this chapter, concentrate on moving slowly and smoothly, breathing deeply and comfortably. Make sure that you relax completely between each repetition. Don't rush. The slower you do these, the more beneficial they will be.

Stretching

Stretching is an important treatment for RSI because of the very nature of the condition. Your tendons and ligaments are foreshortened from scarring and inflammation and need to be gently stretched out. The process of stretching, like limbering, needs to be gentle and slow and is most beneficial when you breathe and relax between repetitions. Everyone has a tendency to hold his breath during exercise. But your muscles need that extra oxygen and the decreased stress that diaphragmatic breathing provides. So remember to focus on your breath every now and again to assure it is slow and steady. Add these helpful stretches to your daily routine as provided by your physical therapist and/or yoga instructor. You can do many of the following stretches at your desk or workstation. Try to make them part of your everyday routine.

Tendon Stretch for Computer Users

- Sit comfortably in an armless chair with your feet planted on the floor.
- Extend your right arm out horizontally in front of you with your palm facing the floor.
- Bend your wrist down so your fingertips are pointed toward the floor.
- With your other hand, gently press your downturned right hand toward your body.
- Press until you feel a pull.
- Hold for about ten seconds.
- Repeat two times.
- Then switch and press back the left hand.

Gradually, as the tendons and nerve compressions ease up in your arm and wrist, this stretch will become effortless. It is a great stretch to do during breaks at the office or at home while watching TV. Make sure you are sitting up straight and your neck and head are aligned with your torso.

Upper-Back Stretch

In a seated position, wrap your arms around yourself as if you are giving yourself a big hug. Inhale and exhale. Relax and repeat two times. Then switch so your opposite arm is on top and repeat the upper-back stretch.

This stretches out those closed, tight upper-back muscles and allows your shoulder blades to open up.

Beyond Limbering and Stretching: The Gym

Your adrenaline is pumping. You've completed your home exercise routine in the mat room and you feel energized but relaxed. You are warmed up. Your brain produces the famous "happy hormone" known as endorphins decreasing the sensation of pain. You feel great.

Everyone around you is sweating as they build their biceps and triceps. Flexing and extending their trapezoids, pectorals, and deltoid muscles in the mirror. You are surrounded by runners jogging in place on the treadmill. You feel as if you can do anything. You are tempted to throw caution to the winds and seat yourself at a Nautilus machine. You are ready to push yourself to your limit. Don't do it.

It's time to apply all that awareness that you've gained from yoga and home exercise routines. The gym can be dangerous or it can be an opportunity for you to increase your efficiency when you move. But there are a few rules you must follow before you begin any exercise in the gym.

• Get your doctor's approval before you begin any gym work.

• If your doctor has given you the green light to work on weighted machines in the gym, *begin with no weight.*

• Take a moment to focus on how you feel. Are you seated comfortably? If you are standing, is your head aligned with your spine? Or is your head thrust too far forward? Take a moment to align yourself and get comfortable.

• Bring a towel with you into the gym. A rolled or folded towel can turn into a wonderful makeshift support if you need a pad on any of the weight machines. When you have RSI, each activity needs to be analyzed with a fresh eye. You may need support or padding where you never did before you were injured.

• Practice each exercise as if in slow motion.

• As you push or pull, focus on how you feel. Do you feel burning, cramping, tingling, sharp pain anywhere? If you do, stop immediately. Stop working on your arms or torso and begin exercising your uninjured legs.

• Pace yourself. If the rest of your day is very busy, you may not want to take advantage of the gym. It may be too much for you. You may instead want to take a hot bath or sauna to relax.

• Remember to breathe as you exercise. You should always inhale when you are lifting, pulling, or pushing. The exhalation happens when you go back to the initial position.

• Don't compete with yourself or anyone else. It is very easy to think that you *should* be able to do three repetitions when, in reality, you are ready only for one or maybe need to stick to the mat exercises for a while.

• Rest between exercises (sets of exercises or exertions). Make a schedule so that you wait at least one to two minutes between each set of repetitions or stretches. Remember, your body is injured.

• Exercise up to your fatigue point but not beyond. Your fatigue point is the point at which you first sense being tired. It may be difficult to identify at first since most of us have spent our lives ignoring it. "I don't have time to be tired" is the popular adage. Before RSI, you pushed through your fatigue to do just a little more. Well, stop it! You are injured now. Learn to recognize your fatigue point and stop exercising. Rest. Walk around. Change activities. Then come back to the exercise when you feel better.

I strongly suggest warm-water exercise if your gym offers such a thing. Many of my patients find water exercise the "turning point" in their recovery. Warm-water aerobic exercise (not swimming, which is too aggressive for most RSI sufferers) works wonders as you are surrounded in heat that relaxes you while you move. The water resistance is gentle and, for most, it is easier to pace yourself in water gravity than on land.

I also recommend taking advantage of a heated whirlpool and/or sauna to revitalize your tired, cramped muscles. Some of my patients do their exercise routines on the mat, then sit in the sauna for a while, and then go and do a few minutes of Nautilus work.

Don't be discouraged. Your strength and muscle tone will return but it will be a slow process. Talk with your doctor or physical therapist about which Nautilus machines might help the most and which machines you should avoid for a while. Remember, once you've been injured with RSI, you are at high risk for a relapse.

The right kinds of exercise combined with good nutrition and rest are pivotal factors in your recovery and RSI pain management. However, total recuperation from RSI requires a multidisciplinary approach. The last step in your journey back to health calls for an in-depth look at pain management. The faster you break the RSI pain cycle, the quicker you will recover.

9. Step Eight: Manage Your Pain

Spencer was an experienced surgeon who was forced to take a leave of absence when some of his fingers became numb. He lost some of the precise control necessary to do surgery and was experiencing sharp, shooting pain in his neck and fingers. Spencer experienced this pain for months before it became too severe to ignore. When he lost some of the motor control of his fingers, he was devastated. When he came to see me, Spencer described his pain and work habits, which involved long hours standing in one position, bending over patients using instruments in small controlled movements. I diagnosed him with ulnar nerve compression, thoracic outlet syndrome, and acute tendinitis.

When Spencer walked into my office, he had deep pain lines on his thirty-five-year-old face. He acted distracted and kept losing his train of thought as he told me about his condition and recent daily routines. Pain had kept him from sleeping through the night for months. He was so sensitive to touch that he pulled away every time his wife reached out. She was confused and angry. He was depressed and scared. Most nights, he moved to the couch just because it was softer and gave more support to his arms while he slept. His pain was disrupting his work and home life. He'd been to other doctors, who misdiagnosed him and told him there was nothing to be done. In the end, even after two years of physical therapy, Spencer was told he would have to live with the pain and dysfunction. He felt his career was finished. Spencer did little exercise or pain management on his own. He didn't know he could help himself break the pain cycle and regain motor control.

You're way ahead of the game. Already you've taken major steps toward breaking your chronic pain cycle and reducing RSI's recurring symptoms. Walking, practicing yoga, limbering, stretching, exercising, and eating a proper diet all contribute to minimizing pain and maximizing your body's natural healing abilities.

The aim of pain management is not necessarily to immediately eliminate pain—although we hope we will be able to reduce it considerably now and cause it to disappear once you have a chance to heal totally from your RSI. Our goal is to diminish pain and help you live a full life while you recuperate. Many of the steps you have already mastered will get you out of bed and moving. They will prevent the muscle weakness that is often so debilitating for those with RSI. But there are no quick fixes. And the bottom line is that *you* have to manage your own pain. Nobody can do it for you. But with the following techniques, it should be a whole lot easier.

Chronic and Acute Pain

There are certain phrases that all my patients who experience chronic pain use, whether their pain has lasted one month or a few years: "Why can't I find relief?" or "I find no real relief." Usually these patients tell me that they have overwhelming feelings of doubt, depression, and despair since they've had this chronic pain. But there is relief to be had both from the physical and psychological effects. If you are experiencing chronic pain due to your RSI, relief is within your grasp. First, we need to understand the physical side of your pain.

Let's look at the difference between chronic and acute pain, their causes and symptoms. Our knowledge of the physiology of pain is not complete, but we do know how pain begins. Pain begins when your nervous system responds to some sort of stimuli, whether it be a punch in the arm, a cut from a glass shard, or another type of injury or disease that causes tissue damage. The tissue-damage message travels by nerve fibers through the spinal cord to the brain, where you "feel" the pain. These pain messages are called *nociceptive stimuli*.

Nociceptive stimuli tell the brain that body tissue has been damaged. The body then reflexively reacts and protects itself. If you've been hit, you pull away. If you touch something hot, you pull back. If you hit your finger with a hammer, you rub it. If you type too long, you rub your hand and wrist—reflexively. If there is bleeding or the damage seems severe, you seek medical attention. Pain tells us to remove ourselves from the source and get help. If we didn't have these messages, we wouldn't try to avoid damage. This kind of pain is called *acute pain* and, despite the suffering it creates, it is an important element of our protective mechanisms.

As you heal from the tissue damage and get treatment, this kind of acute pain eventually fades and your brain slowly changes the message to "everything is fine." But when the pain continues, it may grow worse. Then we call it *chronic pain*. Chronic pain is what we label pain that continues longer than the medical profession would expect a similar condition to last. Usually, *chronic pain* is any pain that lasts longer than three months regardless of its initial cause.

Some of the leading pain researchers have demonstrated that chronic pain is more complex than acute pain but we still don't know why exactly it develops. Nor do we know why some patients are affected by it and others are not. *We do know that many people with RSI develop chronic pain and that the pain is real.*

No Quick Fix

As you may know from your own experience, the frustration level from the pain can grow very high in patients with RSI. There is a strong belief in our society that you go to a doctor to get "fixed." This kind of thinking led one of my patients to have three operations for her various kinds of RSI before she came to me. None provided the relief promised. In spite of this, my patient was still convinced that if she could only have the "right" operation, she would be cured and pain free. When she arrived in my office, she had yet to overcome her belief in surgery as the only cure for her RSI and move on to other options for relief. You and all those suffering from RSI have to take an active role in the healing process in order to stop the pain and begin to recover. You need to consider all options before agreeing to intrusive surgeries.

Sometimes your doctor can become frustrated if your RSI doesn't improve under his care. Without meaning to, he or she may express less sympathy since you may represent his or her own personal failure to provide a cure. You should be aware of this possibility so you can look for a new doctor before you begin to feel hopeless. My coauthor, Ruth, unfortunately, went through this experience during her first two years of RSI treatment. Ruth was dismissed by her first physician with the declaration that "no more could be done" for her. For a period, she felt doomed to live the rest of her life in debilitating chronic pain and limited movement. Luckily, as she recognized her physician's frustration and its effect on her, she recovered her spirits. When she decided his decree was merely an opinion, not a bedrock fact, her options for relief opened up.

Possible Pain Contributors

Pain is extremely complex. When you are in chronic pain from RSI, it is imperative that you dig into your emotions and understand what is going on. This is the only way you can learn to control the various triggers that exacerbate your pain. Only then will you begin to heal. Below are the major contributors to pain that I have observed in my RSI patients.

Anger: You feel rotten and you are spending big bucks as you go from doctor to doctor seeking relief. Your bills mount up as your benefits dwindle. Many suffering from RSI get angry at their condition. If this is you, it is important to understand what you are doing. Anger creates more pain as it causes muscles throughout your body to tighten. The more you can release your angry and tense feelings, the more relaxed and better off you'll be.

Prescription drugs: Many doctors want to offer you relief often in the form of a narcotic, muscle relaxant, or tranquilizer. If you've been on this kind of prescription, your body builds up a tolerance and tries to override the medication's effects. You will find you will gradually need greater dosages in order to obtain the same level of relief. The tension involved in organizing and trying not to forget your next dosage also can set you up for pain as your muscles tense and go into spasm.

The side effects of some of the pain medications can also trigger other conditions. I diagnosed my patient Karen with acute tendinitis in her right wrist and radial tunnel syndrome. Her fingers were weakened and she experienced pain on both sides of her elbow. She had difficulty twisting open jars and doorknobs. Karen had previously been diagnosed by her general practitioner as suffering from clinical depression. She had also just begun menopause. Her internist prescribed a variety of painkillers and an antidepressant. After extensive testing, I determined that in addition to RSI, Karen had fibromyalgia (FMS)—an arthritis-related syndrome that causes widespread musculoskeletal pain—which might have been triggered by her hormonal and depression treatments. Her FMS symptoms only added to her feelings of discouragement and depression. A month later, she developed another condition called compartment syndrome—a painful condition where muscles wrap themselves in spasm around bone, arteries, tendons, and ligaments resulting in severe cramping and acute pain. After Karen's other specialist and I talked, we took Karen off the hormonal replacement therapy and antidepressants. We all agreed that surgery was unnecessary. Karen found relief as the compartment syndrome disappeared. Her depression lifted and her FMS symptoms decreased to almost nothing. The inflammation in her tendons also decreased as did some of the tenderness around her elbow. All of this relief came from discontinuing some prescription drugs.

Karen now lives an energetic, pain-free life. As you can see, it is unwise to treat conditions in isolation. Speak frequently to your doctor about your medication dosage and how you feel. If you sense you are growing too dependent on drugs alone for relief, ask your doctor for suggestions about alternative therapies or read on for ideas I share in this chapter.

Misgivings: As time goes on and your progress is slow, relatives and friends and even your physician, out of their own frustrations and feelings of helplessness, sometimes suggest that your pain may be "all in your mind." You start doubting your own feelings. Is it real pain or am I just asking for attention? Am I going crazy? You may consult a psychologist who, misguidedly, may tell you that you *want* this pain or that you are not thinking *positively* enough to rid yourself of it. You spend more money going to specialists and your pain continues. Mistrusting your own judgment makes every decision more difficult. It doubles the stress in your already stress-filled life.

No matter what happens throughout your RSI recovery, know that your pain is real. You are not imagining it. Trust your body and mind. Don't heighten the tension in your system with second-guessing. Joining an RSI support group may help you air your misgivings among an open, understanding audience and release stress that otherwise might build up and worsen your condition.

Disuse: As the pain continues, you find you want to rest more and more. Your muscles become flabby and your movements more and more inflexible and limited. Your bones, too, lose calcium as you avoid activity. Decreased or restricted activity can actually alter your body's fluid balance, electrolyte balance, both local and general circulation, and can cause muscle "wasting" from loss of nitrogen. These weaknesses create other secondary aches and pains, which may help you conclude you need more rest. Don't succumb. Walk and stretch regularly.

Self-image: Although you look healthy to everyone around you, you have begun to see yourself as disabled from RSI. You have no self-esteem. You describe yourself as a person in constant pain. You are depressed and apathetic. You see no hope, no future, no options. You may want to seek help from a psychiatrist, psychologist, or counselor.

The common way to address all of these is to realize your *beliefs* are wrong. Chronic pain is not the same as acute pain. *Acute pain* is often helped by pulling away, resting, and taking medication. For relief from chronic pain, you require a multifaceted, long-term plan like the one outlined in this book. When you are frustrated or angry, read through this section again for added support. You are on the right track to recovery.

Taking Action Against Pain

RSI patients and others who suffer from chronic pain have to *learn to interpret the chronic-pain messages* differently from acute-pain signals. Chronic pain does not stem from a new injury and your actions should be different from those you employ when you are first injured. Here are questions to ask yourself to help you understand and resolve chronic pain.

1. Have I just worked too long and not taken enough breaks?
2. Is this pain a signal to rest and stretch?
3. While moving, did I extend beyond my comfort zone (the posture or position before pain is triggered)?
4. If I have been resting, am I resting too long? Do I need to walk and stretch out those spasms and pressure points? Do I need to apply ice and heat to reduce the flare-ups of inflammation and increase mobility?
5. Is the exercise or technique I am using correct? Did I lift my arms too high? Where am I holding tension while I exercise? Is the angle of my neck triggering pain in my hand?

Adjust Your Attitude

If you can adjust your thoughts and beliefs to include the following ideas, you will start to become aware of how you move and how you relax, and use both to manage your pain and heal.

- I will concentrate on how I think and *feel.*
- I will work carefully, always being aware of when my pain begins and when it ends.
- I will not be afraid.
- I will be patient with myself

To beat RSI, you really need to learn to move differently. You need to teach your muscles to move while relaxed so there is no reinjury. You must also work to banish bad habits of awkward positioning, bad posture, and no rest breaks. Your RSI is a sign that you have worn down muscles in your body. They will no longer function in the way you have become accustomed to using them. It is time for a healthy lifestyle that involves becoming more self-aware. An added bonus to these changes is that they will make you a happier and healthier individual. Even when you no longer have chronic pain, you must maintain your newly developed flexibility, strength, and movement range as well as your heightened self-monitoring awareness. You need to be *muscularly aware* or you will wind up injured once again.

Raise Your Muscular Awareness and Decrease Your Pain

Muscular awareness begins with your breathing. You have already practiced diaphragmatic breathing in the three chapters about breathing, yoga, and exercise. It is just as important for you to be *breath-aware* whenever you experience pain.

Many RSI patients live in fear of their pain and, unconsciously, tense their muscles and hold their breath throughout daily activities. Are you doing this? If so, you are aggravating your condition. To help your body heal, pay attention to your breathing throughout your day. Relax and trust yourself. Be willing to feel your muscles as they move once again. When you find yourself holding your breath or becoming tense, consciously will yourself to relax and breathe deeply. This will quickly release your muscles so they move freely. You may be surprised at the amount of relief you feel from practicing this one exercise regularly.

One of my patients, Sally K., who was in chronic pain for six years before finding relief, swears that her whole world changed when she stopped holding her breath. "I'd find myself holding my breath when I was putting away the dishes. This simple task is always extremely difficult and painful for me. The minute I began inhaling and exhaling as if I were limbering—I could feel my muscles relax. I also felt better because I was making the job easier and less painful for myself. I then stopped pushing myself past my pain line. I figured out easier ways to stack the dishes and take more breaks. But the breathing is what made me aware of what I was doing to myself."

Relieving Painful Muscles

There are many different ways your muscles can hurt. When you understand why your body reacts the way it does, it is easier to know what to do to relieve the pain. Below are the different kinds of muscular problems you may have and some suggestions on how to relieve the pain in each case.

Muscle spasm occurs when a muscle contracts strongly and won't let go and is often accompanied by a sudden, intense pain. A spasm may limit or prevent movement altogether. RSI injuries often involve tight muscles that are apt to spasm around the upper spine and neck. When you turn your head and a sharp pain radiates down your arm and up your head—that's a muscle spasm. Heat packs or a warm bath often help relax the muscles and release the spasm.

Muscle tension is the result of an unconscious tightening of the muscles. When someone has a headache, his brows furrow as a result of muscle tension. I often notice that my RSI patients unconsciously hold their shoulders higher than is normal, which is also a result of muscle tension. There are many ways to release this tension. The limbering exercises in chapter 8 can be extremely effective. Yoga, massage, hot packs, and exercise also can be helpful in easing tight muscles in your neck, shoulders, arms, and hands.

Muscle weakness is the condition that often underlies both muscle tension and spasm. Unfortunately, it seems to be a condition of modern life. Many patients I see are weak because they don't exercise or they spend too much time in one position usually seated in front of a computer screen. Their muscles weaken out of disuse and become vulnerable to arthritis and RSI. If this lack of exercise or static work conditions sounds familiar, you may be developing muscle weakness. Exercising, even if it's only for forty-five minutes a day, will help you improve your general health and prevent injury. You should also take regular breaks at work and use them to stretch and revitalize those tired, strained muscles.

Trigger points are nodes of degenerated muscle tissue that, when pressed, send pain throughout the immediate area. They usually develop in the wake of prolonged muscle spasm or tension. Many of my patients with RSI develop trigger points. Trigger points can be treated with cortisone injections right into the muscle, followed by special physical therapy. Be sure any injections you have are done by a specially trained doctor who is highly experienced in this area.

Fibromyalgia (FMS) is diagnosed when a patient experiences eleven or more painful trigger points (sharp, throbbing muscle pain and soreness) throughout the body. FMS often accompanies long-term RSI. Although diagnosis of FMS is still a challenge, physicians use the following as guidelines and diagnostic criteria to indicate it in a patient: Pain must be present in the neck, front of the chest, middle or lower back, and shoulder or buttock for each involved side. Widespread pain must be present for three months. Why it often follows or accompanies long-term RSI is unknown. Distinguishing FMS from RSI is usually done by determining the multiple trigger points that are not usually indicative of the RSI condition. However, many of the same factors exacerbate fibromyalgia and RSI such as fatigue, lack of sleep or restless sleep, physical exhaustion, and a sedentary lifestyle.

Inflammation from both FMS and RSI seems to respond to fish-oil supplements, bromelain, and quercetin. Exercise, usually walking, is also often prescribed for both conditions; however, those with RSI can start with much longer walks and progress more rapidly while FMS patients should start with five-minute walks and increase them by only a minute each week until forty-five minutes is reached. Human studies using six tablets daily (1,200 milligrams) of magnesium malate—a combination of magnesium and malic acid—have also shown this to be extremely beneficial for those with fibromyalgia. This combination does not seem to exacerbate the symptoms of RSI. (Consult your certified nutritionist and doctor before beginning any supplemental regime.)

Inflammation, Strain, and Pain

Other RSI factors contributing to pain are inflammation and strain. A common culprit is tendinitis, which can be a small tear or inflammation of the tendon that often takes a long time to heal. Tennis elbow, a condition that causes pain on the outside of the elbow due to inflammation and strain, is another common injury under the RSI umbrella. Repair begins in both conditions after the inflammation subsides (about four to ten days). In about two weeks, a tendon callus forms along with adhesions, which are the undesirable fibers of collagen that attach to the lining of the tendon. As you would imagine, adhesions restrict the movement of the tendons. Muscular weakness from these adhesions puts force on the joint and often arthritic changes result in knees, shoulders, or wrists. Unlike pure muscle pain, ligament and tendon damage regain strength through passive motion exercise—your physical therapist will gently move your arm for you during the exercises. This kind of exercise speeds up healing and prevents adhesions. Limbering exercises and rest will also help to strengthen the damaged area if done slowly and without any force.

I am not going to discuss the many anti-inflammatory drugs or muscle relaxants on the market as they would create a book in themselves and I am not a strong proponent of them in most cases. There are, however, excellent resources that you can consult for more information on them. (See the Reading List at the back of the book.) I will caution you as to the possible side effects of most anti-inflammatory drugs. Many of these drugs can eat away at the lining of the stomach and result in ulcers and other digestive disorders like irritable bowel syndrome. I strongly suggest that you discuss preventive medical treatments with your doctor before beginning any pharmaceutical regime. If you do, one of the most effective preventive over-the-counter products I've come across to protect your stomach lining is liquid acidophilus (lactobacillus acidophilus [LA]). Acidophilus comes in both capsule and liquid form, but if you've been taking lots of drugs, use the liquid as it is more quickly absorbed into your system and will work faster. (It is suggested that you keep the liquid form refrigerated after opening.) Taking just a few teaspoons per day will keep the chemistry of your stomach balanced and replete with the proper "friendly" flora necessary for good digestion. LA and bifidobacteria are examples of these friendly floras that grow in the gastrointestinal, urinary, and vaginal tracts. Because they are "good" bacteria, they control the bad bacteria and prevent them from overpopulating the human system. Studies suggest that LA and other friendly flora may protect a person from colon cancer.

Your stomach needs lots of protection while you are dealing with pain. Gastritis is sometimes attributed, among other causes, to eating while emotionally upset. Yeast infections are also said to be triggered by tension.

Getting Away from a Painful Lifestyle

Estelle was a freelance journalist and going through a particularly bad period in her life. She felt frantic as she tried to hide her RSI from her various employers, fearing that they would hire other writers if they were afraid she couldn't meet the newspaper's deadline. She supported herself and didn't feel like there were any options except to push through the pain and continue the hectic writing schedule that had brought on her RSI. Her friends tried to help but they had their own lives to deal with and the amount of help she needed day to day increased with her pain level. I finally convinced her to try some of the techniques recommended in this book. On one of her visits, I was thrilled to hear that she had started focus walking. I then showed her how to set up a schedule for rest periods while working on an article. She invested in a voice-activated software program that allowed her to speak her thoughts into the computer. And she kept bags of ice in the freezer and a heating pad ready to help with especially hard days. She posted diagrams of exercises she could do while resting at her computer. We set up a "hand budget"—the time she could use her hands before pain began—for her major activities and added the necessary time to complete each task. With all this organization done, Estelle's stress decreased. She felt more in control and her depression began to lift.

All this helped. But the real change came when her attitude shifted. Once Estelle understood that her highest priority was her own health, her life began to fall into a saner and more relaxed lifestyle. As a result, the quality of her work improved because she could now concentrate better. Her pain began to recede as she slowed down and began to heal. After Estelle approached her editors to discuss her needs, they became more flexible about her assignments. The deadlines remained, but she was given more lead time to research and write her articles. Estelle found her healthy lifestyle, stopped reinjuring herself, and is pain free today.

Another patient of mine recovered much slower. Molly was newly married. Severe RSI symptoms began acting up about three months into the marriage. Her doctor recommended that Molly stop working immediately. She and her husband were very worried about money even though he had a secure, high-paying job. But they decided she could stop work for a while. They could financially manage it. However, both Molly and her husband missed the main point—they still didn't understand the reason she needed to stop working. She needed to stop using her hands and shoulders in stressful ways. Instead, they both viewed her time off as a minivacation and an opportunity for Molly to do all the household chores they had both been too busy to accomplish. As you can imagine, Molly's condition worsened. When pain prevented Molly from doing her chores, her husband began to resent her "princesslike" attitude. He felt unfairly burdened suddenly with a house and wife to support. He had envisioned a partnership when he married. Now it seemed as if he was doing a list of chores when he got home after a hard day at work while his wife sat and watched, ordering him around. His wife felt guilty, and was bored and frustrated. He was frustrated and angry and they began to take it out on each other.

Many of my patients tell me their partners respond the way Molly's husband did. This is partly because RSI is invisible and easy to forget if you are not personally experiencing the discomfort. But the extent of fear and denial in a couple can also be strong. In Molly's marriage, neither she nor her husband was willing to believe the extent of her injuries and accept the changes that needed to be made in order to stop the pain and prevent permanent damage. Happily, Molly and her husband finally went into counseling and began to work through some of their individual and joint fears and concerns. But because of their denials, Molly's recovery was delayed over a year. When each individual in a partnership gets behind the recovery process, it will happen faster and the relationship usually becomes stronger.

The Unfairness of It All

RSI is not fair. No one plans to be injured. And, sadly, no one is invulnerable to life's inequitable surprises. I see too many patients ignore their needs, like Molly, because, even in relentless pain, they unconsciously believe they will get better if they just ignore this discomfort. Here's a fact for you: If you ignore RSI, you can become permanently disabled. If you ignore the pain, you may never be able to lift, pull, hold hands, sleep, or walk without constant pain. Don't do this to yourself. You are worth more than that. You can't afford to ignore your pain. Address it today and start on the eight-step road to recovery.

Supplements That Accelerate Healing and Reduce Pain

Proteases are enzymes that chew up protein. They work in digestion, cell division, cell replacement, and more. The proteases travel to injured sites to control inflammation and promote healing. Supplemental proteases are backups that help natural proteases do their job better. There is encouraging clinical evidence to support the use of protease supplementation.

• In several studies involving patients with injuries, 90 percent of the subjects had less pain, swelling, and redness after taking protease supplements. Plus they healed faster and returned to their normal activities more quickly.

• A group of people with severely sprained ankles were given protease supplements. They experienced less pain and swelling and were able to move around better than the group with similar injuries who didn't take the supplements. The protease group returned to work in 1.7 days whereas the control group returned to the office in 4.4 days.

• At the University of Pittsburgh, football players found that their minor injuries healed faster when given proteases compared to injuries of placebo-treated players. Proteases have been found effective in aiding recovery from sprains, strains, surgery, and digestive problems in hundreds of scientific studies. The pharmaceutical companies document the proteases' anti-inflammatory benefits in acute injuries. They are true anti-inflammatory agents and are safe. They have been used for over forty years by millions of people. Besides being anti-inflammatory they also enhance the healing process. They are noted to be one of the best nutritive healers for severe injuries, including joint injuries.

However, if your RSI has moved into a chronic stage, proteases will probably not help. Proteases are best used as soon after the injury occurs as possible. This is sometimes difficult to determine with RSI as it is a cumulative injury. But if you end up needing surgery, take the proteases one or two hours before surgery to hasten your recovery. These supplements don't "store" in the body and become ineffective if the injury is three or more days old. You can take five to ten tablets at a time. (Check the bottle.) For best results, take the supplements on an empty stomach with water or juice (not milk as it will interfere with protease activity and absorption.) Continue to take the protease four times a day about thirty minutes before meals and bedtime. Continue for seven days or until healing has occurred. Select a protease that is enteric coated—this protects your stomach lining by resisting stomach acid. Protease combinations of trypsin, chymotrypsin, bromelain, and papain have been found to be most easily absorbed by the body and thus are the most effective types available.

If you are forced into an activity where you know there will be excessive wear and tear on your injuries, protease supplementation may help to protect you. Obviously, the best idea is to walk out of the situation. But we all slip occasionally. If you know you will encounter a highly strenuous and stressful period, proteases might help with the resulting inflammation and irritation. It is especially effective with the two chronic conditions tendinitis and tenosynovitis.

Protease is found in many sources including pineapple (bromelain is the supplement), papaya (supplement: papain), aspergillus molds (fungal vegetarian proteases), and hog pancreas (trypsin/chymotrypsin and pancreatin). Before taking any supplement, I suggest you consult your doctor.

A Word about Painkillers

In my years of practice, I've noticed the adverse side effects of pain-killers usually offset their benefits for many of my RSI patients. However, if you find that you and your physician decide drugs are the appropriate approach to address your pain, use them only for the short term and only when all your other options are gone. The group of painkillers most often prescribed, either over-the-counter or from the druggist, is called NSAIDs (nonsteroidal anti-inflammatory drugs). These include Advil or Motrin (ibuprofen), Naprosyn (naproxen), and Feldene, to name a few. I stress using these only for short-term relief because these drugs tend to build up in the body over time. Even the newer NSAIDs block the formation of prostaglandins and can become toxic if you take them too long. Taking ibuprofen for a headache once in a while can't hurt you. But RSI chronic pain sufferers tend to take more and more of these painkillers, which can work against them in causing severe damage to their joints and increasing the pain. It is impossible to know who will have a bad reaction to these drugs as everyone has a different safety threshold. But potentially, NSAIDs can damage cartilage, the liver, kidneys, the stomach, immune system, bone marrow, and the nervous system. Aspirin has been known to destroy cartilage and block its repair as well. This can speed up the progression of any dormant osteoarthritis. The gastrointestinal problems associated with NSAIDs are alarming. They range from stomach ulcers and hemorrhage to perforated ulcers.

Other Options for Pain Relief

Hot and cold packs: As I mentioned before in chapter 3, one of the most effective ways to reduce the inflammation and muscle spasms and increase flexibility is the alternating use of hot and cold packs. Always begin with the cold, which reduces the inflammation, and then apply the heat, which increases your circulation and relaxes the muscles.

Corticosteroid injections: Injecting corticosteroids directly into the joints supplies immediate yet temporary relief of pain, stiffness, swelling, and inflammation. I suggest you question your doctor closely about alternative treatments as this is not one I recommend. In the 1950s, there were human studies that indicated that steroid injections caused long-term joint damage and suppressed the adrenal functions. They also found that, in the long run, the injections could damage tendons.

Other injections: Injecting anesthetics (such as Novocaine) dulls the pain so that you can move and perhaps ease a muscle spasm. I have seen the effectiveness of this method before acupuncture or physical therapy. The area in spasm is dulled so that the other therapy can reach and relieve the real problem. This fairly benign process is relatively painless and has no side effects. Many of my patients have temporarily benefited from an anesthetic injection.

Relationships and Pain Management

Remember those promises made at the altar: ". . . in sickness and in health; for richer or poorer . . ."? Well, RSI will really test the mettle of any relationship you are in when it strikes. I strongly suggest counseling if you get into trouble emotionally. The entire dynamic of your relationship shifts when one person is injured. That delicate balance of independence and financial security comes into question as you and your partner feel a new vulnerability. Being ill brings up complex issues that you may have never openly discussed with one another. An objective third person, such as an experienced counselor, may be just the ticket to keep you both together and open in the face of the challenges RSI can introduce.

The sudden sense of loss as you lose your ability to use your hands is frightening for you and your family. There are many situations in life that merit some outside help. We can't be experts in everything. As you learn to deal with this change in your life, you will grow and learn to communicate your needs and be more sensitive to the needs of your loved ones. You will heal faster in a positive, supportive environment. Chapter 11 addresses these problems in greater detail and offers more solutions to some of the problems you may be facing at home.

The Value of Distraction

Everyone has heard the joke, "I went to the doctor the other day and said, 'Doc, I have this awful headache.' 'No problem,' answered this wise physician. 'I have just the thing.' Wherein, he proceeded to stomp heavily on my foot. 'Ouch!' I yelled in amazement and shock. But miraculously, my headache vanished. Now, only my foot hurts."

Obviously, you should not take this joke literally. Spraining your foot will not help your upper-body RSI. However, another type of distraction will help you. Sitting around and brooding will only intensify your pain. When you begin to view your injury as your business, this boredom will begin to dissipate. One of the biggest problems for those with RSI who have to leave work is isolation and boredom. Your isolation will lessen as you walk to your appointments, make an effort to meet with friends, work with others, improve the work environment, and educate others on RSI prevention and treatment techniques you've found to be effective. If your mind is very busy, it doesn't have time to "hear" those pain messages. Laughter, relaxation, social functions, and manageable jobs all help. Make a list of all the activities you enjoy and people with whom you like to socialize. Try to integrate them into your week. I've seen time and again that patients who make an effort to care for themselves dissolve their pain more quickly and completely than those who don't.

Your Sense of Humor Is a Pain Killer

"Mature laughter is the playfulness of one who has experienced suffering but has not been conquered by it." Patty Wooten, R.N., in her book *Compassionate Laughter: Jest Your Health* (Commune-A-Key Publishing, 1996), explains the value of adult humor. Humor helps us let go of our restricted view of our environment or our situation. When you have RSI, humor is your best friend. Laughter is the best stress reliever, your finest muscle relaxer, and the greatest distraction you can ever find. Laughter allows us to detach ourselves from our problems and from our pain.

Laughter is a cathartic cleansing that can wash away our anger, frustration, and animosity. I wish every RSI support group would put together a list of videotapes and audiotapes that make each participant laugh. Too often I find that the one thing never shared in the groups is humor.

We know that stress is a necessary part of life—stress actually promotes balance in our bodies. Without stress our skeletons could not maintain an erect posture. The tension of opposing muscles balances them. Exercise puts stress on the cardiovascular system. Eating puts necessary stress on the digestive system. But it is the prolonged stress and strain, like that resulting in a repetitive strain injury, that creates the emotional response "fight or flight." We, and all animals, respond in "fight or flight" when we perceive a threat to our lives, according to Harvard physiologist Walter Cannon. RSI results in the third stage of stress, what Cannon calls exhaustion. This is where stress-related diseases and injuries develop.

Humor and laughter can be an antidote to this harmful kind of stress. A sense of humor helps us feel we are in control of the emotion. It helps us create a positive emotion from what appears to be a negative event. RSI is serious, but the stress that created the environment for the RSI to flourish needs to be dissipated. During your RSI recovery, go out of your way each day to laugh hard at least once. You won't regret it, I promise, and you'll forget your pain if only for a moment.

Other Therapy Options

Here are some tips as you explore different therapy options.

• Don't let your eagerness for a cure lure you into trouble. Ask the practitioner about his training and experience.

• Ask about the cost over the phone as you discuss your first appointment. Many insurance companies still won't cover anything beyond physical therapy. You don't want to be surprised financially.

• Be wary of any practitioner who is not willing to work with your regular doctor. Give him the boot! All your health-care practitioners ideally need to work as a team. You may run into a primary physician, however, who doesn't believe in any alternative treatments. In that case, use your own best judgment. Relief is your goal regardless of the shortsightedness of some of your practitioners.

- When evaluating their diagnosis and treatment suggestions:
  —ask how the conclusion or plans were reached
  —ask if the conclusion is based on theory, hypothesis, or other scientific proof
  —give yourself time to think about and digest information before agreeing to treatment.

The Food and Drug Administration (FDA) prints free publications to help educate consumers about the maze of new treatments. To receive a free FDA publication, send your name and address and item number(s) to Consumer Information Center, Pueblo, CO 81009. The pertinent item names are Choosing Medical Treatments (Item #537C) and Unproven Medical Treatments Lure the Elderly (Item #546C).

Body Work and Massage

Body work and massage treatments provide many benefits. You can refer to chapter 3 for an in-depth discussion of these treatments. You may want to talk to your doctor about the many different types of body work and massage available to:

- enhance body alignment
- reduce swelling, inflammation, and muscle spasms
- increase the flow of oxygen and blood in the body
- boost flexibility and range of motion
- diminish pain
- help speed recovery of soft-tissue injury.

Deep-Tissue Techniques Successful with RSI

We already discussed the benefits of one deep-tissue technique, myofascial release, in chapter 3. Below are other methods that have proven effective for some RSI sufferers.

Rolfing: This is one of the most famous deep-tissue body-work techniques that concentrates on structural reintegration, or realignment, of the musculoskeletal structure of the body.

Philosophy: Proponents believe that the vast majority of muscular aches and pains are the result of tension caused by a structural imbalance. Pain begins when the connective tissues become so "solid" that they begin to constrict nerve and neuro pathways.

Over a period of time, we lose the ability to relax those muscles at will. Tense, contracted muscles not only lack any "give," they lack an adequate supply of blood and oxygen thereby trapping the body's toxic metabolic wastes. We feel stiff and achy when this happens.

Another contributing factor, already discussed, is the musculoskeletal discomfort called "gluing." This occurs when your connective tissues adhere to each other thereby limiting your movement. Because you have to work harder against the stiffness and immovable tissue, you feel weary. Movement becomes an exercise in fighting your own body.

What happens when you are Rolfed? Ida Rolf discovered a way to release the adhesions and contractions of the body over time. The Rolfer will do this in a carefully orchestrated sequence of ten sessions focusing on each major muscle area and gradually covering the entire body. By skillfully applying slow, steady pressure—a deep-tissue massage with traction and stretching—Rolfers are able to release the offending contractions, thereby restoring muscle ease and bone position and reestablishing balance and flexibility. There is occasional discomfort since the massage is so deep, but many have found the long-term results worth it.

The end result: The end result of Rolfing, according to its proponents, is that the body moves and feels "well oiled." Musculoskeletal aches and pains, like those symptomatic of RSI, are either greatly reduced or eliminated. Leon Fleisher, a prominent classical pianist disabled by RSI thirty years ago, is a strong proponent of Rolfing. He reports that Rolfing techniques helped him to the point that he is now making a cautious comeback as a pianist using both hands. In a *New York Times* interview, he stated that ". . . Rolfing has been stretching my muscle fibers that haven't been stretched for thirty years. It is a manner of manipulating connective tissue, and it looks like a deep massage in slow motion." (*The New York Times*, 1 November 1995.)

Hellerwork: This technique is not as well known as Rolfing, but its proponents claim it to be equally successful. Hellerwork assumes everyone is healthy and it is used to treat chronic pain and to help "well" people learn to live more comfortably inside their bodies. It combines deep-tissue muscle therapy and movement reeducation with counseling about the emotional issues that may underlie a physical posture. Participants go through eleven sixty- to ninety-minute sessions. Its focus is on alignment by stretching and manipulation of connective tissues called fascia.

Movement Integration Techniques

These techniques emphasize posture and alignment—perfect for correcting harmful habits that can exacerbate or cause RSI. They also teach more efficient ways to use damaged joints or achy muscles so that movement and balance take less effort. These movement therapies are considered safe and the best way to find out if one might help is to try it. You can expect to feel more stable and to move more freely after learning the various techniques. Many of my patients, after finishing a number of Feldenkrais or Alexander sessions, feel they can now do other exercises such as tai chi or yoga with much less pain.

The Alexander Technique emphasizes the integration of the entire body in order to solve a specific problem. For example, practitioners of this technique believe that if you have a back problem, the most effective way of resolving it is to become aware and thus be in control of the supporting musculature of the back. Both the Alexander Technique and the Feldenkrais Method emphasize eliminating unnecessary muscle tension and harmful postural habits that cause and prolong pain. The Feldenkrais Method, besides addressing postural habits, focuses on heightening awareness through movement using a specific series of lessons. These lessons make you more aware of your limits and movement needs during your everyday life and help you make healthier choices as you move. Both the Alexander Technique and the Feldenkrais Method believe that the act of becoming aware of *how* you move actually makes changes in the ways that you move. Since both disciplines have proven to be extremely beneficial to my patients with

RSI, I suggest you observe classes in each technique and decide which approach you prefer.

The Feldenkrais and Alexander methods involve teaching the individual ways to move that more naturally fit his skeletal and muscular structures, thus reducing stress and strain. Instructors teach simple, efficient physical movements designed to improve balance, posture, and coordination, and to relieve pain. A session may focus on movements as basic as getting up from a chair properly or discovering how to move your arm comfortably without triggering pain. In both disciplines, the instructors go through rigorous years of training before certification is granted.

The Trager method: The Trager method combines light tension-releasing massage with a series of gentle, painless, passive motions that help individuals expand their range of movement and release muscles. The Trager method is, in general, less practiced than either the Alexander Technique or the Feldenkrais Method but it can be surprisingly effective. It relies a great deal on gentle shaking and vibrations. The therapist can, in effect, cause confusion of the muscles so they relax or "let go." The muscle doesn't know to "hold on" because the shaking has disturbed the neural signals coming through. This is sometimes combined with myofascial release methods and has optimum effect.

The Healing Arts

Acupuncture has been studied and used by the Chinese to cure soft-tissue injury for over five thousand years. Many of my patients have found it highly effective for reducing inflammation and swelling and temporarily blocking pain giving the body a chance to use its natural resources to heal itself.

The *traditional acupuncturist* places hair-thin needles called filiform needles at specific points along which energy flows throughout the body. Only about fifty vital points along the meridians of the human system are used for common ailments even though over eight hundred have been identified. "These needles inserted at vital points along the meridian network are used to stimulate, sedate, accelerate, block, and otherwise modulate the intensity and flow of these energies," states Daniel Reid in his *Shambhala Guide to Traditional Chinese Medicine*. Once these energy points are modulated and balanced, the body can function at its optimum level for health.

In *electrically enhanced acupuncture*, the practitioner places the short, hair-thin filaments at vital points on the meridian of the body or injury site. Then gentle electronic stimuli, similar to a TENS unit, is attached to the protruding tips of the filament needles. You should feel no discomfort from the needles and only a dull pulsing sensation from the electronic stimuli. The electrical impulses "root out" the pain, reducing the inflammation and naturally enhancing the body's abilities to heal itself. Many of my patients have found electrically stimulated acupuncture effective for muscle release and for breaking the pain cycle. I can personally recommend this approach. It does not work for everyone, but it is extremely effective for some.

It often takes a few sessions of acupuncture for the swelling and inflammation of an RSI injury to recede. The long-term effects of acupuncture therapy vary with the individual. I've seen the technique break enough pain cycles and allow enough patients to finally get a good night's sleep to suggest you try it. Acupuncture also blocks the neuro pathways that tell your brain that you are in pain.

Acupressure and shiatsu: Shiatsu means literally "finger pressure" in Japanese and refers to the Japanese form of acupressure. Both acupressure and shiatsu are used to treat deep-tissue bruises and arthritis pain and are often combined with other massages when treating RSI. Shiatsu involves the application of varying degrees of pressure on the various 660 trigger points of shiatsu zones. Patients have reported moderate short-lived success with these methods of pain control and muscle-tissue release. They are best when combined with neuromuscular massage.

Mind-Body Group of Therapies

Disciplines such as biofeedback, mental imagery, autogenic training (autosuggestion and imagery combined), hypnosis, and quiet meditation have all been proven effective in reducing stress and controlling pain. However, patients with extreme symptoms of RSI may have difficulty following the quiet immobile routines necessary for these approaches to succeed. You may find it easier to meditate while focus walking and to practice mental imagery while stretching and limbering. If you are interested in trying these disciplines, discuss with your physical therapists how to comfortably use each of them.

I have obviously not included all the alternative therapies available for pain management and healing from RSI. However, the disciplines discussed above are the most successful that I have seen thus far when treating my RSI patients.

Pain-Management Centers in the United States

A multitude of pain-management centers have cropped up all over the United States in the last few years. Pain management has become big business, and with this development comes many new options from which you can choose. Before you decide to enter into treatment at one of these centers, ask your doctor for a reference. There are a couple of core philosophies and approaches that you can ask about.

1. Drug-oriented pain-management centers. I recommend you stay clear of these since I don't believe that drugs ultimately relieve chronic pain. If the doctors in charge of the center have strong pharmaceutical training, that might be your first clue as to their orientation.
2. The holistic approach: I tend to favor this kind of eclectic approach where the center's physicians and therapists look at how you move, your lifestyle, as well as your particular injury site. These centers are especially effective when treating RSI. The centers' philosophy and disciplines may vary widely from myofascial release and needle trigger point therapy to Rolfing and other forms of deep-tissue massage. A center's director should be more than willing to explain his center's philosophy and approach to you before you decide to begin treatment.

C. Everett Koop, M.D., former U.S. surgeon general, wisely advises that in the terrain of alternative medicine, there is no prescription more valuable than knowledge. I believe that applies to both the traditional and alternative areas of medicine. Information gives you back control over your health. It lowers stress, and helps you heal faster. If one therapy doesn't work, try another one. Pain management is difficult when you have RSI because you are usually dealing with a combination of injuries and a lifestyle that needs some major changes. The steps in this book should help you develop the answers that fit your specific injuries and life changes. Traditional and alternative medicines are your tools to help you heal. Please use our healing program to empower you on your journey back to a healthier life.

PART II

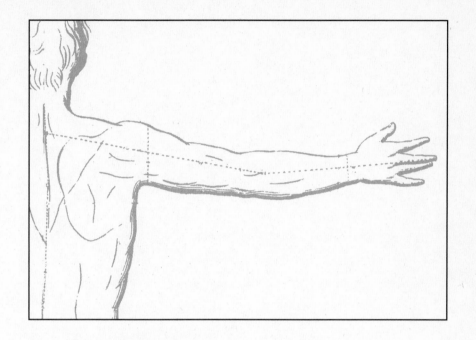

Special Concerns—Women, Office Ergonomics, Housework, and Intimacy

Introduction

Now that you are using the eight-step program, it's time to look beyond treatment. Part 2 introduces you to some of the special issues concerning women who have RSI. This section offers suggestions about easier and healthier ways to continue being a lover, friend, and housekeeper while you are recovering. Two people were involved in the creation of this book. Part 1—the eight-step healing program—was told from Dr. Simon's point of view. This next part is from my perspective.

I am Ruth Aleskovsky, a polio and RSI survivor, a former sign language interpreter, and a medical writer. I had polio as a child, which affected my legs and spine. I was forced to relearn how to walk five times in my life. The coping skills I picked up from that experience have proven invaluable. I used them in my successful struggle to overcome RSI, which I got as an adult triggered by overuse of my hands as a sign language interpreter. I suffered from a severe case of RSI for over six years. I was told by more than one doctor that I would not recover and would remain in chronic pain for the rest of my life. I am happy to report that with the help of Dr. Simon and his eight-step program, my symptoms disappeared. I am today pain free and healthy.

During this period of recovery from RSI, I totally rearranged my life to decrease my pain and increase my comfort. For example, I got a voice-activated computer to save my fingers from typing, brought pillows to the cinema to support my injured arms while I sat, and bought a food processor to minimize chopping in the kitchen. I asked for help and suggestions from everyone around me during those years. I did not keep my condition to myself. I told friends and family about my limitations so they could help me overcome them.

I knew from my polio experience that each new environment demands different angles of approach, pacing, and range of movement to insure comfort. Each new chore presents a new challenge when you have RSI. The simple tasks of carrying a package, shaking a hand, or opening a door require reeducation of what were once reflexes. When you are healthy, you adapt to new experiences effortlessly. When you are injured, especially when your upper torso and limbs are involved, a single new experience requires conscious planning in terms of movement, emotional adjustment, and time management. I know how exhausting it can be just to get through the day with RSI.

As I questioned others who had RSI about problems facing them at home and at work, I heard too many comments similar to those that I had made when I was looking for relief from RSI pain. People had the same complaints and were often coming up with the same answers but didn't know it, while others entirely overlooked the solutions. A book such as this one was obviously needed. Someone had to collect and share the best tips and suggestions about coping with RSI and everyday chores.

In addition, I noticed that no other book covered the special problems that we women who have RSI face. So I spoke at great length with a leading gynecologist/obstetrician about the various issues that complicate or distort diagnosis and recovery for women. I also interviewed leading experts about cutting-edge ergonomic technology that will help the RSI community stay productive and healthy.

This section is the result of my personal experience and additional research. I hope it will provide you with helpful hands-on approaches to solving your everyday problems as a sufferer of RSI. Read it carefully. It was a labor of love, and, I hope, it will help improve your life.

10. Women and RSI

I compiled this chapter from hours of interviews with women who have RSI, leading gynecologists and obstetricians, and piles of research articles. It solely addresses women and their unique issues when, along with perimenopause, pregnancy, osteoporosis, mastectomy, and menopause, they face RSI.

Kay was diagnosed with RSI five years ago. She followed her doctor's treatment advice to the letter and was able to keep her job as an editor. She was recovering and feeling great. Then Kay noticed a lump on her right breast. Soon afterward, she was diagnosed with breast cancer. She agreed to a procedure, a lumpectomy, in which four malignant lumps were removed.

Suddenly, Kay's right shoulder and arm became inflamed and all her RSI symptoms returned twofold. She was forced to take a medical leave because of all the pain and weakness she was experiencing. Kay's doctor reexamined her and found she had developed a double-crush situation—the ulnar nerve was compressed in two places under her arm. As a result, Kay had almost constant numbness, tingling, and loss of sensation in this area. Some of her motor control was also gone in her arm.

None of her doctors—all specialists in RSI—made the connection between her cancer surgery and her recurrence of RSI symptoms. Luckily, Kay decided to do some research herself and ultimately discovered a link between her two conditions in some case reports in a medical library on the Internet. Some tingling and muscle atrophy was, in fact, due to her cancer surgery. When Kay shared her new information with her RSI doctor, he reviewed her surgery records and changed her treatment. He suggested a surgery that would relieve the double-crush condition. This new surgery technique was appropriate now that he understood which symptoms were due to her cancer surgery and which were due to her RSI condition. Because of perseverance and a strong belief on Kay's part, she is almost pain free today.

Kay's case is not unique. Most Western doctors are specialists. It's difficult to find someone who has the more holistic focus of Eastern medicines. Too often, Western doctors only concentrate on the body part or illness connected with their specialty. When I was diagnosed with RSI, no one informed me that I was already at high risk because I had had polio. I was trained at an early age to push through the pain and live with it. I also unconsciously compensated for my polio-weakened legs with my strong upper-body muscles by often making them work twice as hard. I probably would have recovered more quickly had I been aware of these facts when I was first diagnosed with RSI. Dr. Simon, the third doctor I consulted, was the first doctor to mention polio. The human body is too complex to compartmentalize its ailments and influences. Many wonderful physicians are aware and do suggest alternative treatments to their patients. Nevertheless, some still ignore the fact that their patient's hormonal changes can aggravate her RSI symptoms.

Women have more and different conditions that may exacerbate symptoms or trigger an earlier onset of RSI than men. Luckily, most doctors are all too happy to learn something that will help their patient. Often, it is a well-informed female patient who starts the questioning that results in the recognition and dual treatment of more than one condition. The information here will help you be aware of the questions and concerns to raise to get the best care and treatment for total recovery.

Premenstrual Syndrome

One woman with RSI had this story to tell. Does it sound familiar?

> I felt like I was going crazy. I tried to take care of myself—not
> do anything that obviously aggravated my RSI symptoms. But
> every two and a half weeks, like clockwork, my RSI symptoms
> would worsen. My whole upper torso ached, my arms throbbed,
> and my fatigue worsened. What I figured out was that the
> increased pain coincided with my premenstrual time. I got smart.
> I avoided caffeine and chocolate—though I craved both—food
> that would aggravate my RSI symptoms during my two "good
> weeks." I kept exercising even when I didn't feel like it and did
> lots of cold and heat contrasting arm baths. Most important, I
> stopped beating myself up. I actually had convinced myself that I
> was hurting myself consciously, although inadvertently, every
> time I felt pain. When I understood how hormones, nutrition,
> and exercise were related, I began to relax. I added deep relax-
> ation and yoga to my routine. Gradually, the PMS and RSI symp-
> toms stopped interacting so much and I have not only lessened
> my pain but now feel more in control.

Even if you rarely experience premenstrual syndrome (PMS)—
cramps, headaches, mood swings, water retention—your RSI symptoms
may become worse during the one to two weeks before the onset of your
menses. According to Dr. Sharon Diamond, a leading New York gynecologist, the cause for this primarily hormonal change is a rise in your
progesterone level. Progesterone is the ovarian hormone that promotes
the continuation of pregnancy. This progesterone increase affects your
muscles by creating the elasticity (laxity) in our joint connections that
women need during pregnancy. It allows the pelvis and surrounding
muscles to become more elastic and expand to adapt to a growing fetus.
During pregnancy, then, you may find it easier to move your joints.
That's the positive side.

Overall, progesterone is no friend to women with RSI. When this
hormone increases, it often generates painful muscle spasms. Water

retention, common during PMS and pregnancy, only adds to the pressure on our already compressed nerves and tendons and can even result in bloated hands and arms. Already swollen and inflamed soft tissues become even more sensitive and painful during this time of the month. Ask your physician or physical therapist for specific exercises to help relieve the discomfort of your PMS period. Judith Lasater's book, *Relax and Renew: Restful Yoga for Stressful Times* (Rodmell Press, Berkely California, 1995), has easy exercises that are RSI safe and may help relieve PMS symptoms.

Here is what else you can do:

• *Pamper yourself and don't panic*. You are not having an RSI relapse. The increase in discomfort of your RSI symptoms may decrease when your menstruation begins.

• *Your discomfort will last only for a short time*. Even if you have none of the classic symptoms of PMS, your body still produces more progesterone during the two weeks before you menstruate. This may be why your RSI symptoms become heightened temporarily.

• *Remembering the cause* and temporary nature of the increased pain alone may help you cope with the discomfort.

• *Ask your therapist for special exercises* and your doctor for advice about reducing water retention.

• *Drink six to eight tall glasses of water daily*. Water is the great equalizer. It flushes out the unwanted extra toxins and helps you absorb the nutrients and minerals you need to heal.

• *Avoid caffeine, chocolate, and soft drinks*. Calcium is an important factor when fighting muscle spasms and the cramping women often experience monthly. The calcium levels in most women's bodies decrease during premenstrual periods. The carbonation in soft drinks can block calcium absorption. Caffeine and chocolate are stimulants that can also trigger muscle tension and spasm. However, if you are one of the many women who craves chocolate during her menses and you must indulge, *here is a tip: Freeze a Milky Way or Snickers bar*. Frozen chocolate is just too cold and too hard to chew quickly or in quantity. It prevents all except the most determined of souls from bingeing.

• *Pay attention to calcium and iron* during and right before menses. Levels of both often decrease during menses. Ask your physician if you are a candidate for supplements or if you should work on your diet to assure that you are getting enough of these nutrients.

• *Keep exercising.* The more you exercise, the less chance your muscles will go into spasms, the more vigorous your circulation will be, and the better you will feel. So exercise wisely and gently. Even slow, moderate exercise will benefit your struggling body.

Following the above advice should help drastically reduce your PMS symptoms and RSI pain during your premenses period. Give it a try.

A *research note:* At one time, it was held that vitamin B_6 deficiency was part of the reason for the monthly progesterone rise. Neither B_6 nor any other supplement is known to help moderate progesterone at this time.

Pregnancy

Pregnancy is another time when progesterone shoots up. Pregnant mothers commonly complain about swollen ankles and hands during their nine months. If you have RSI and are pregnant, you may feel increased pain, tenderness, and numbness during your pregnancy. However, this is still a new area of research (pregnancy and RSI symptoms), so don't assume your RSI symptoms will worsen when pregnant. Some obstetricians report that their patients' symptoms actually *decrease* during pregnancy. Science doesn't have an answer about why they decrease—yet.

Research also shows that women are sometimes prone to develop carpal tunnel syndrome during their pregnancy. Apparently, one of the places a pregnant woman retains water is in her wrists, which puts pressure on and constricts the carpal tunnel. If you did not have carpal tunnel syndrome until you were pregnant, consult your obstetrician about appropriate treatment during this time. You need to take care of the symptoms and be assured the condition will end one or two months after the birth of your child. Your body is going through so many different changes during pregnancy that monitoring all of them for your comfort is vital. Consider this just another aspect of your pregnancy.

Perimenopause and Menopause

Again, wide fluctuation of hormones occurs during perimenopause and menopause. *Perimenopause* is the few years before *menopause*—the time when your period naturally ceases—when your period may become irregular and you may experience irregular monthly menses. Both menopause and perimenopause bring on natural hormonal fluctuations, which can cause mood swings, hot flashes, and a change in your sleep patterns. These hormonal changes may aggravate your RSI symptoms as well. If your RSI symptoms have increased and you suspect a hormonal link, talk to your doctor about steps you can take to reduce the added pain and inflammation. To date, however, research has not proven that these changes *initiate* RSI, as pregnancy can.

We need more research to answer our questions about what happens to our bodies during these periods. Specifically, we need to discover what impact a woman's RSI condition has on the rest of her system. One hopes that gynecologists will start asking questions and RSI specialists will begin looking at a woman's entire system and interactions.

Diet and Nutrition for Women

Most of us want to eat right, but we don't want to give up all the goodies. When we don't feel well, we crave comfort food and therefore it can be a challenge to eat only what is good for us and our RSI recovery. When I asked a few doctors about the optimal diet for women, their answers surprised me. None of them felt as if science was really clear yet on what an optimal diet is. Overall they agreed that a diet low in fat that includes lots of fruits and vegetables, more complex carbohydrates, and fewer processed foods is a good idea. They all also emphasized that women usually need more calcium than they can get from their daily diet.

When I asked about sugar and, even more important, chocolate, I was thrilled with the response (being a devout chocoholic myself). The doctors explained that an occasional piece of birthday cake isn't bad for you. Only people who have difficulty metabolizing or who binge on sugar should abstain. However, as Dr. Simon points out in chapter 6, sugar can create mood swings and rob your body of the nutrients it needs to heal. More than the occasional piece of chocolate may heighten the risk of slowing your recovery process.

Salt can cause water retention; therefore, use it in moderation. If you are prone to PMS, it may help to avoid salty foods right before your period. Salt also may increase blood pressure for some. If you find you have high blood pressure and salt seems to trigger it, avoid it. Use other spices for flavor enhancement.

Osteoporosis and RSI

Osteoporosis is a disease in which the bones become extremely porous, are subject to fracture, and heal slowly. The main cause is insufficient calcium. During our forties when we are fully mature, we start to lose more bone than we regenerate. Our bones become progressively more porous and brittle. In people who develop osteoporosis, the bones may deteriorate at a faster-than-normal rate.

To give you an idea of the scope of this disease, osteoporosis causes 1.3 million fractures every year and costs the nation more than four billion dollars in medical costs. As you can see, this is a very serious disease and one for which women should be checked regularly after they begin menopause. Although not exclusively a "woman's" disease, more women than men are diagnosed yearly with osteoporosis. Forty thousand deaths annually are attributed to this condition. Educate yourself so you can take care of yourself and practice prevention.

Treating Osteoporosis and RSI

Osteoporosis makes RSI worse, and RSI worsens osteoporosis. When a woman's calcium absorption rate decreases, her hormonal balance shifts, making her particularly vulnerable to osteoporosis. RSI patients with osteoporosis require a carefully integrated and well-directed rehabilitation program, according to Dr. Simon. Their treatment plan should include a slowly progressive exercise regimen that considers both painful disorders.

Many women with osteoporosis have painful conditions like RSI or arthritis that were diagnosed after osteoporosis and which may interfere with their ability to exercise. When a woman develops RSI as a secondary condition to osteoporosis, she may have a strong tendency not to exercise because of the severe pain generated by both conditions. She is more prone to be sedentary and often won't want to move because of her discomfort. This only compounds the problems in both conditions. Exercise will relieve the pain and build muscle and bone mass thus offering relief from the discomfort of both conditions.

We know that lack of exercise leads to a widespread dysfunction of the body's systems, or *systemic dysfunction*. Cardiopulmonary insufficiency, progressive weakness, and muscle atrophy can occur. This vicious cycle of increasing pain and progressive deterioration is all too common with the combination of RSI and osteoporosis.

If you suspect you may be facing RSI and osteoporosis, you should start by getting an accurate diagnosis of all your conditions. Unfortunately, most patients are well into their painful syndromes when their RSI is diagnosed. But easily adaptable treatment programs for women with both conditions are available. Massage, yoga, and physical therapy can offer great relief. Multidisciplinary approaches, including these therapies, were unheard of five years ago. Today, Dr. Simon reports that many doctors integrate new therapies with an incredible success rate when treating RSI and osteoporosis.

Walking is also beneficial to patients with RSI and osteoporosis. A great healer, it improves each condition with no negative side effects. Exercise with weights is highly recommended as well for those with osteoporosis as the bones respond by becoming stronger. When RSI is severe, weights can be used on the legs; gradually, as the RSI heals, more weight-bearing exercises can be added using the arms.

Osteoporosis also causes a thinning of the bones. When the bones become thinner, stress increases on the joints and other parts of the body. This added stress will aggravate your RSI symptoms, weaken your joints, and slow the healing process. Talk to your physician about extra vitamin supplements to slow the bone-thinning process and speed up your recovery time. Here are more reasons for those with RSI and osteoporosis to exercise:

• **Weight-bearing exercise makes the bones respond by becoming bigger and stronger.** Walking with light leg weights, climbing stairs, and standing exercise bicycles with back rests are great for both conditions. Be careful with the weights. If you notice that they alter your posture or cause your gait to be unbalanced, you may be straining your injured limbs. Discuss the best approach with your physical therapist.

• **Exercise increases the flow of blood** to the bones and muscles thereby increasing the availability of bone, muscle, and tissue-enriching nutrients.

• **Exercise stimulates electrical currents within the bones, which stimulate bone growth.**

• **Calcium supplements only work with exercise.** They do nothing to strengthen your bones without exercise. The calcium will flush right through you without the stimulated blood flow you get from exercise.

• **Walking and yoga are great for both RSI and osteoporosis.** Make sure you discuss your conditions with your yoga instructor so that she or he can modify the postures and prevent straining your weak or injured limbs.

• **Warm-water aerobic exercise** is good for the joints and all your RSI needs. Water lessens the impact on your muscles and joints, and the warmth relaxes your muscles while you move. However, the water does not provide enough resistance to keep your bones strong. Consider combining land and water exercises to complement both of your conditions.

How to Enhance Calcium Absorption and Fight Osteoporosis

• **Exposure to sunlight** usually provides adequate vitamin D, which allows your body to absorb calcium. Of course, moderation (a half hour per day maximum) is the key as the sun's ultraviolet rays are no longer friendly to our skin and can cause skin cancer when skin is overexposed. This doesn't mean you need to cower indoors. Use a sunblock and you should be safe.

• **Eat foods containing lactose** (milk sugar). Most dairy products provide both calcium and phosphorus. Some physicians suggest you drink three glasses of milk or ingest at least eight hundred milligrams of calcium daily. More than that may lead to excess phosphorus, which can limit calcium absorption.

• **Avoid aluminum- and magnesium-based antacids.** You don't need the extra aluminum and magnesium that are often found in antacid products. Read labels to avoid any products that contain aluminum and magnesium. When you ingest too much of these two minerals, they can cause increased excretion of calcium. That's not bad by itself but this increased calcium excretion will cause too much phosphorus to be excreted from your bones as well. When too much phosphorus is in your system, all the lovely excess calcium is reduced so your body won't have a sufficient supply. When your calcium/phosphorus ratio is unbalanced, you can become very ill. Your body doesn't easily get rid of aluminum and, in addition, research shows a link between excess aluminum and senility and the probability of developing Alzheimer's disease.

One Woman's Story of RSI and Osteoporosis

Denise worked as a legal secretary for twenty-five years. She worked in a typical RSI high-risk setting—long hours, few rest breaks, lots of coffee and cigarettes. She skipped too many meals and got too little sleep.

Denise described her first warning of trouble as her "bad winter." Usually a highly accurate typist, she began to make lots of typing mistakes. Her left hand felt numb and no amount of shaking or massage helped. When Denise saw her doctor, he diagnosed carpal tunnel syndrome and sent her to physical therapy the following week. On her way to physical therapy, she slipped on a patch of ice and broke her ankle in two places. When her doctor looked at her X ray from the emergency room, he said it also revealed the beginning of osteoporosis. Denise said, "It was too much all at once. I was angry. It was unfair. I had to laugh at myself after I threw one whopper of a tantrum in my poor doctor's office. He was sweet, though. Gave me time to cool off and then we got down to business. I went on a special diet with an extra calcium supplement. I started exercises that helped both my hand and foot. The hardest thing for me was quitting smoking. But I did it. My ankle took a long time to heal but, when they removed the cast, I did exercises in warm water. Both my hand and ankle healed over time. The long-term goal I have is to learn how to be more patient with myself. It's hard but I think I can do it."

Cancer and RSI

Don't Skip That Checkup!

Whenever you are injured, your immune system has to work overtime to heal, and, therefore, it is more susceptible to other diseases and illness. Many women are tempted to skip annual gynecological exams when they have RSI since their schedule is already filled with doctor and therapy appointments. I interviewed an alarming number of women who did just that because they were burned out and couldn't face another exam of any kind. Remember that this is the time to take extra preventive care of yourself. Breast cancer statistics are sobering, striking one out of every ten women. The incidence of cervical and uterine cancer is also high. But, thankfully, as women learn to take advantage of mammography and other means of early detection, the incidence of all these cancers has started to decrease. Don't skip your gynecological checkup and forfeit your advantage against cancer for anything.

Mastectomy, Lumpectomy, and RSI

If you are diagnosed with RSI, and you've had a lumpectomy or mastectomy, it is important to mention this to your doctor. The surgery can trigger a relapse of your RSI symptoms as it did in the case of the next woman. "The scar from my biopsy was small. The doctor had removed the lump and given me a clean bill of health. I had completely recovered from RSI the year before. A couple of nights later, my RSI symptoms recurred. When I consulted my doctor, he looked at how I was using my arm. He asked if I was doing anything differently since the surgery. I couldn't think of anything. Then he asked me to show him how I sat when I drove. So, I sat down and pretended I was driving my car. He asked why I kept my right arm draped over the seat. I told him that it was more comfortable and something I did without thinking. When I stopped draping my arm, the swelling and tenderness disappeared. I apparently was compensating unknowingly for some scar tissue in my breast when I draped my arm. I feel fine now."

According to research, when a woman has a mastectomy or dissection under the arm to remove lymph nodes, she may develop *armadema*—an arm swelling. This type of surgery can exacerbate, if not initiate, the onset of upper-extremity RSI. Armadema may or may not set in depending on how many nodes are removed, how deep the cuts, and the level of the surgeon's skill. If you have a lumpectomy, biopsy, or mastectomy, please discuss this with your RSI doctor.

Women who have had reconstruction surgery after cancer surgeries often have excellent results. However, sometimes radiation damage occurs that may not become apparent for up to twenty years later. Consequently, there may be stiffening, hardening, and, sometimes, swelling of the breast tissue. We don't know why the damage can lie dormant for so long but clinical histories show that it can. If you have RSI, such an inflammation and inelasticity of tissue can further weaken muscles and aggravate your symptoms. If you have had cancer surgery and now have RSI it is a good idea to ask your RSI physician to review your surgical records. What he will be seeking is data concerning the depth of the surgeon's incisions and the number of lumps removed. This will greatly help him in his diagnosis and treatment plan.

Remember: Any kind of surgery makes an area more susceptible to a cumulative, overuse injury like RSI. Be sure your physicians communicate and share records so you can get the best treatment and quick relief.

Coping Strategies from RSI Women

This chapter is all about being more aware of everything that may be happening in our bodies. Raising our consciousness so we are sure to think of all the possible links as we consider RSI treatment and talk with our doctors is no small feat. But I believe women know that a good patient is one who addresses and deals with all aspects of her health.

As I interviewed women for this chapter, I heard about many common-sense strategies that were the pivotal reasons individuals began to feel better from RSI. Some were obvious. Some were not. I incorporated some of their suggestions into my RSI coping strategies. I hope they help you with your recovery.

What follows are some ideas and feelings from women who have successfully managed their RSI:

• "I went to a nutritionist and discovered lots of food that aggravated my RSI symptoms and which food would give me more energy, especially during my period. I discovered that oysters were chock-full of calcium (I could live on oysters!) and canned salmon had more than four hundred international units of vitamin D (I love salmon patties). I was in seventh heaven. This diet isn't so bad after all."

• "When I finally understood *when* my symptoms get worse, it really helped. I was able to plan my time better and take care of myself more effectively. I knew what to expect. I was more in control."

• "I started to dress in looser, warmer clothing. I stayed away from salt and soda. My PMS and RSI symptoms decreased."

• "The hardest thing was to convince my various doctors that they needed to take the time and talk to each other. Once they finally did, they came up with anti-inflammatory medicine I could take days *before* PMS began. It was amazing how much each of them didn't know about the others' specialty."

For resources where you can access medical research and get information about various conditions specific to women, see the Internet Resources section in the appendices.

11. The Ergonomics of Living: Setting Up Your Home and Office

According to the Occupational Safety and Health Administration (OSHA) more than 700,000 workers are afflicted with RSI each year making it the fastest-growing category of workplace injuries in the country. Everyone agrees that the way your desk or office space is set up can mean the difference between working comfortably and suffering aches and pains—or worse. Gradually, we are becoming more and more aware of the importance of a healthy workspace with computers, assembly lines, and other machinery. Still, we humans have a lot more to do besides business. We have work to do in the home. Most of us do laundry, dishes, bed making, dusting, and vacuuming at one time or another. Beyond these issues of daily work, there is the simple task of getting dressed—something you probably did almost unconsciously before suffering from RSI. Now you not only struggle with the machines you operate daily, you are also having trouble unbuttoning your favorite shirt or blouse at night. Let's first take a look at options for creating a healthier office space and then we'll go on to home solutions.

A Short Review: RSI and Work

Static work, like computer work, obstructs free blood flow and upsets the body's natural protection from lactic acid poisoning. As you've seen in the first part of this book, blood flow cleanses the muscles, metabolism continues, and you are spared fatigue and strain. When you sit all day, this natural invigorating and cleansing process is interrupted. The blood vessels within the muscles are squeezed for as long as your muscles contract and if you don't take a break and relax, the blood flow is drastically reduced to your hands and arms for long periods of time. When your posture is also static, your neck and trunk muscles can contract thus decreasing the blood flow through your body even more. When there isn't enough blood flow, nutrients and oxygen metabolically change and begin to generate a toxic lactic acid buildup. Sitting all day just doesn't provide enough blood flow to get rid of that toxic waste, and you begin to feel aches and pains and fatigue. That's why taking breaks is so important. Change positions while you work, walk around, and let that blood flow! Remembering what is happening to our bodies as we work and changing those bad habits is the only way to prevent RSI, promote health, and keep our jobs. Also, if you can explain clearly to your supervisor why you need to take a break and walk around, he or she is more apt to understand. Your extra breaks will become a way to maintain high productivity and not be perceived as a vehicle to "slack off." Keep this in mind if you are working through your RSI recovery.

The most familiar upper-extremity RSI is carpal tunnel syndrome. It is the most carefully defined and studied of all the nerve entrapment syndromes in the upper extremities. RSI is rapidly increasing as the American workplace is flooded with computer terminals. The Department of Labor estimated in 1994 that more than forty-five million U.S. workers used computers each day, although many of them spent the majority of their work day on other tasks. The hours of computer use and reported incidence of RSI has doubled today with eighty million workers filing RSI workers' compensation claims in 1997 alone.

Poor ergonomic environments are the common cause of excessive strain on the soft tissues and are responsible for the onset of carpal tunnel syndrome and other kinds of RSI. Let's look at them and how you can decide what to change for your benefit.

Setting Up an Ergonomically Friendly Office Space

You have a computer, a printer, and maybe a fax machine in your office. Where should you put them for the easiest, healthiest access? What kind of chair should you get and where should your lights go? A well-designed space can reduce your risk of injury by promoting comfortable movement and reducing the strain of daily repeated activities. Consider how your body relates to your furniture and machines and think about how the machines relate to each other. The right decisions can simplify your life in the office. Here are some suggestions on how you might think of arranging your office components.

Your Chair

There are a wide variety of chairs from which you can choose. And they are not all expensive. Remember, too, that expensive chairs are not always better for *you*. What is good for your neighbor may be ergonomically wrong for you. How do you know what's good for you? There are a few parameters to bear in mind when buying a chair. Make sure you can adjust the height of your chair. When determining your daily chair height, keep in mind your feet should ideally be flat on the floor with your elbows and knees forming something close to right angles when your hands are on the keyboard. If you feel some lower-back stress, try a low footrest for relief. Place a cushion between your lower back and the chair to support the lumbar regions where your back naturally curves. You should also be able to adjust the chair's arms to rest your forearms on them without slumping or hunching your shoulders. When you sit in your chair, relax, don't slouch, and get into the habit of changing positions periodically. Vary your tasks if you can and take frequent, short breaks to stretch, stand, and walk. You can install software programs to remind you to do this or simply use an egg timer.

Your Desk

You should have enough room on your desk for your monitor, keyboard, and a document holder. The document holder supports papers or books at a comfortable height for you to see while typing. These holders can attach to your monitor or stand on your desk. It's important, as you know, to move your head while you are working so your neck doesn't get stiff and trigger inflammation. These document holders give you a comfortable "other" place to look while working at your computer. The space on the desk should also be deep enough to place your monitor at a comfortable viewing distance, which is about arm's length for most of us. The desk should be high enough not to touch your knees or thighs and your legs should be able to move comfortably beneath it. Avoid awkward unnecessary stretching and twisting by placing things like your phone, fax, printer, and teacup within easy arm's reach.

Your Monitor

Your monitor should be at eye level or slightly below so you don't have to tilt your head back or down when you are looking at it. Keep the monitor clean and use an antiglare screen to improve screen contrast. If your monitor is too low, there are inexpensive monitor stands you can purchase at your nearby office supply store. This stand may also free up more desk space for you. If your monitor is too high, raise your chair and use a footrest if your feet are then not flat on the floor.

The Two-Monitor Advantage

If you have neck problems from your RSI, try these suggestions made by my ergonomic consultant from the Mount Sinai Technology Rehabilitation Unit. I have incorporated all of them into my workplace, and they have provided constant security against neck pain for me. I have a laptop and another monitor set up. In this way I can use both monitors at once giving my neck lots of movement and forcing my whole body to move slightly. This prevents static positioning, which, as we know,

YOUR EYES

You have two goals: avoiding glare and keeping the light in the room balanced. You can minimize glare by controlling light sources in the room or by placing your monitor at a 90-degree angle to the window or other bright light. To balance the light—so your eyes don't tire from constantly adjusting to different light levels—keep overall overhead lighting lower when you're working with a computer than you would when reading a newspaper. Use a focused task light to illuminate documents you are copying.

Remember to blink. Staring is a kind of overuse syndrome itself. Computer users forget to blink, making their eyes dry. Get regular eye checkups. If your eyeglass prescription is incorrect you may be leaning toward your computer to see, causing back, shoulder, and neck strain. If you do a lot of copying or referring to documents, the optometrist can give you bifocals that will help you see both screen and paperwork. If you are stuck at a computer all day, take eye breaks by looking off into the distance. The following wonderful yoga eye exercise eases sore and twitching eyes. It strengthens the eye muscles that are often underused and relaxes the overused ones. You can do this refreshing exercise at your desk without anyone noticing and stay healthy. If you wear eyeglasses, remove them for this exercise. Do not attempt this exercise if you are wearing contact lenses.

The yoga eye exercise:

• Sit comfortably with your head, neck, and back aligned in a straight line, your feet flat on the floor.

triggers RSI strain and pain. I also have a window to the left of my station so that I can gaze outside across the city to rest my eyes and give my neck another position to try. With the addition of voice-activated software, I am able to both stand and sit while working. This constant change in position allows me to relax my whole body.

Ergonomically Correct Equipment

Something is only *ergonomically correct* if it fits you personally. If your company is trying to accommodate your workplace in light of your present injury, work with them. Occupational therapists and ergonomic consultants can make very helpful suggestions. But you are the only one who can determine what is comfortable for you. Your whole body has

- Fix your gaze straight ahead at a spot on a far location, such as a wall or building out a window. Then close your eyes.
- Take a few deep breaths and relax.
- When you open your eyes, focus again. Keep your head still as you do the following movements.
- After each cycle, close your eyes and relax.
- Inhale and look at the ceiling without moving your head.
- Exhale and slowly move your eyes clockwise. Count each number on your imaginary "eye clock" as you pass it.
- When you reach six you should be looking down at the floor, your head still steady.
- Inhale as you move your eyes back up to twelve.
- Keeping your head relaxed and perfectly still, circle the eyes *counterclockwise* using the same breathing technique.
- Close your eyes and relax.
- Repeat three times.
- Then rub the palms of your hands together until you feel heat.
- Place the cups of each palm over your eyes. Feel the heat relax the eyes and their muscles.
- Put your arms down. Relax and take a deep cleansing breath.

Tip: If you feel dizzy or feel any other discomfort, stop immediately, close your eyes, and relax.

to say yes before it is *correct* for you. Try everything before you buy and check to see if you can return the piece for a full refund if it doesn't work out.

Wrist Rests

Wrist or palm rests are firm padding that is placed snugly in front of the keyboard. Their benefit is controversial. Some experts say wrist rests will reduce strain on the shoulders as computer users can rest their wrists on them instead of holding their arms in the air while keying. And other specialists claim that wrist rests prevent free finger movement and actually aggravate RSI. If you decide to use wrist rests, the height of the pad should allow you to maintain your wrist at its natural keying angle while working. If you feel any strain at all, eliminate the wrist rest immediately. Personally, I think they create awkward angles that can cause more damage than help. Ergonomic experts suggest that you type with your wrists flat, don't bend them up or down, and let them float over the keyboard. Armrests can help support the elbows. Most importantly, when typing, try to relax and don't pound the keys.

Footrests

Footrests are not necessary for everyone but can add comfort if there is a mismatch between your body size and your office furniture. They can make all the difference in the world to a desk worker with short legs or a high chair. When your feet are grounded, there is no pull of gravity, you feel more stable, your muscles relax, and you feel more comfortable. In this way, footrests prevent foot and leg fatigue and promote better posture that will help fight general weariness and overall strain. They are now sold at the big office supply stores or can be ordered from one of the catalogs in the appendices.

The Document Holder

Document holders hold papers and books upright so they can be seen comfortably while you work. Sold at office supply stores, these holders are an inexpensive investment that can prevent neck and back strain since they prevent you from bending to see documents. They are really excellent ergonomic aids that, research tells us, actually improve productivity by making it easier to work. Position your holder upright. You can find some that rotate vertically and laterally to change the distance as needed. Some sit on a pivot arm so you can position them near the monitor and the keyboard. The simple upright holders are inexpensive and lightweight. You can move your chair closer or move the holder nearer to you.

The Ergonomic Keyboard and Mouse

There are so many different ergonomic keyboards and mice that finding and buying the right one for you can be confusing. Again, the design of these tools is important, but *the determining factors are in how you sit and use them.* Recovering keyboard athletes need more than a "hand-friendly mouse" to get through the work day. There are several kinds of ergonomic mice on the market: one design has a thumb rest on one side, another incorporates a track ball, another uses a joystick to release those cramped arm and hand muscles of yours.

The only way to choose a new keyboard and mouse is either to bring them back to your office to test for several days or go into a store and test the products there. If you decide to order the product and test it in your office, make sure the manufacturer has a thirty-day money-back guarantee. It is worth your time and effort to get the keyboard and mouse that is easiest and safest for you to use.

Your Phone

If you use the phone often, you should consider getting a speakerphone or headset. Cradling the phone between your neck and shoulder contorts and cramps your neck and shoulder muscles. There are a few headsets with and without their own phone systems on the market that are reputed to have especially clear sound with little or no feedback.

For noncomputer use, two companies make headsets that are superior to other products on the market today: Plantronics (1-800-544-4660) and Hello Direct (1-800-520-3311). Both plug into your phone system and are exceptionally clear. They plug into any phone handset. When I have been on the phone with people using these systems, I couldn't tell that the user was wearing a headset. There was no echo and no feedback. But try several to see which fits your phone system best. These systems are sturdy and good for everyday use. Plantronics ships worldwide and has a special-order division. If you need a unique modification built, they will do it—for a price, of course. Each company has different return policies. They are usually reasonable, but it is important to know exactly what the policies are before you buy. Tapetel Electronics (1-800-228-1751) sells most brands of headsets and can help you through all the technical compatibility problems. They will also assemble the system for you before shipping if you are unable to do it yourself.

Voice-Activated Software

This is software that enables you to speak into a microphone and see your words instantly typed on the screen. It is perfect for busy workers who don't want to learn to type. It is also ideal for the recovering RSI keyboard user. The software controls the mouse and can do everything you usually use your hands to do on the computer. It was originally invented for those without any hand use (quadriplegics and others with little or no motor control). Now it is also being used by a much larger group for its convenience.

If you are using IBM's NaturallySpeaking voice-activated word processing program, VXI Corporation (1-800-742-8588) makes a phone headset with something they call the parrot switch box. The parrot switch plugs right into your computer. If you need to use the phone while you are working at the computer, you just press the switch and your headset (the same one you use for voice-activated software) will switch to phone use. The negative with this equipment is that the switch is very delicate and is easily broken. But the tone is clear and it is easy to use.

Here are some safety tips I found helpful while using my voice-activated software program:

• *Always keep a tall glass of water nearby.* It is alarmingly easy to overuse your vocal folds (cords) and wind up with a hoarse voice or, worse, injured cords. Keep your throat and cords moist and happy.

• *Move around while you work.* Some of the software on the market demands that you constantly watch the screen as it gives you choices as to which homonym or other word you want typed. This can intensify a tendency to maintain a static position at the computer. Remember to move and take frequent breaks. With a long microphone cord, you can stand, kneel on your chair, and sit as well as shift in your seat.

A newer addition to the Dragon system (IBM's voice-activated software) is the Dragon NaturallySpeaking Mobile. This is an RSI sufferer's dream come true. So many times, we are in situations where we want to jot something down so we don't forget. This is a light tape recorder that you can speak into while away from home or the office and then attach right to your PC on your return. It quickly converts your recorded speech to text without your touching a keyboard. It is advertised for "busy people everywhere" cutting out the need to schlepp your heavy laptop to a meeting. Unlike the Dragon Dictate, you don't need to keep your eyes on the screen when the program is translating your speech to typed format. You *will* have to reread your copy once it is typed. The system has a correct button on it. You simply highlight any word that needs correcting, and, like Dragon Dictate, you will be given a list of five words from which to choose. IBM has many showrooms, and they would be happy to let you try it.

The hitch: This mobile recorder only works with Dragon NaturallySpeaking word processing software. You can cut and port it to Microsoft Word but it slows the recognition time down and works better with NaturallySpeaking. Minimum system requirements are a Pentium processor, 266 megahertz and at least 64 megs of ram. However, for instantaneous recognition (less than half a second), IBM suggests 96 to 128 megs of ram. If you are thinking of using this on a notebook or laptop, I suggest you visit IBM's Web site at www.DRAGONSYS.com where it will tell you which machines are compatible and which are not (the voice card has specific requirements that all mobile units don't have).

But if you can get the machinery to use this stuff, do it. It's a great help to all who have RSI and can be used after recovery to reduce the possibilities of relapse.

Easing RSI Pain at Home

The office isn't the only place you use your arms and hands. After a long day at work, you go home to face more handwork. Keep in mind that simple things you do can help you reduce your stress and ease the strain on your injuries. Let's look at the *possibilities* instead of all the *can'ts* that have been enveloping you at home. The trick is to break down each chore into small, easily accomplished steps with lots of rests in between. You must figure out how to execute each step with the least amount of pain and pain-triggering movements. This may take some experimentation on your part given your height and size and degree of RSI.

However, the following suggestions should help you create the solution that is right for you. They should provide you with the tools and the mind-set to once again learn how to do these household chores effortlessly as you retrain your muscles to work differently. Let's get started.

Opening Doors

Since doors are a problem at work and at home, this is a good place to face the dreaded doorknob. Pulling weight after a simple twist of the wrist as you do when opening a door is painful and sometimes simply impossible with RSI. Here are suggestions on how to overcome the KNOB.

• For less than a dollar, you can buy grip liners sold in kitchenware shops and supermarkets. Traditionally, these liners are used between stacked china plates to prevent slipping and scratching. For RSI sufferers, they provide relief whenever you face a door. Keep one of these squares in your pocket or purse and when you come to door, wrap the liner gently around the doorknob. It will do most of the twisting work for you. You only twist your hand, wrist, and arm minimally when you use these squares. These are also great to have in the kitchen for opening jars or picking up bottles. Buy a few and always have one handy.

• You can also use the stronger parts of your body instead of your injured arm to open the door for you. Ask your physical therapist how to do this in one of your first sessions. Pull the door open just enough to stick your foot into the opening. Then roll your hip in to open it further. Your torso follows so the weight of the door rests on your strong back, which can open it the rest of the way with ease. Once you learn this effortless and pain-free technique, you'll never go forward through another door.

Then there are doors that are just too heavy to move. When you encounter these, I suggest you wait until someone comes along and opens it for you or call security or the person you are visiting for help. Doors are exhausting and we tend to go in and out what seems like hundreds every day. Perfect these adapted ways of opening doors and you will save yourself tremendous energy, effort, and pain.

Breaking Down the Task

Regardless of your stage of recovery or stamina level, you need to break down each task so that you rest *before* any pain is triggered. As you limber each morning, the exercises should remind you of your comfort zone for movement range, your hand budget (the length of time you can use your hands before pain begins), and, of course, the importance of breathing while you move. When you are first attempting a task, I suggest you rest every five minutes, regardless of whether you think you need it or not. Use a timer set for five-minute intervals to alert you when it is time to rest. This will prevent your wily mind from convincing you that because the task is familiar and was easy (before RSI) you can do more if you just do it fast.

These frequently spaced rest periods will make your progress slow. However, believe in pacing and in giving yourself more time than you expect you'll need. Accept the reality that you may not complete the task in one session. Your recovery depends on your willingness to give your body the rest it needs to heal. Keep this in mind when you feel the tendency to speed up or skip a rest period.

Laundry

Laundry is a perfect task to *break down*. Here are some suggestions on how you can reorganize your laundry and do it in a timely, painless manner.

• **Detergent:** Get yourself a couple of light (one cup) plastic containers. Scoop out (or pour if you use liquid detergent) enough for one load of laundry. Do the same for bleach.

• **Buy a small cart:** Use this cart to transport the laundry to and from the laundry room whether your machines are in or out of your home. These carts do vibrate, which can aggravate your sensitive arms, but the bother is much less and using them is more handy than trying to lift a bagful of laundry. Obviously, if you have stairs in your home, you may want to transport the laundry by hand but in small bundles instead of trying to drag a cart up and down the stairs.

• **Dirty-clothes sorting:** You may already sort your laundry into colors and white loads. If not, you can avoid the tedious and often tiring task of sorting by having separate laundry bags dedicated to each laundry load and, when full, just empty the entire bag into the washer—no sorting necessary.

• **Do a little at a time:** Try to do the laundry before it accumulates or use a small cart to move the laundry. Do only one kind of laundry at a time (dark or white.) You will find trying to do too many loads will trigger lots of pain.

• **From washer to dryer:** The movement of putting laundry in, and especially taking it out after it's washed and still wet, can be almost immobilizing to RSI sufferers. If you can't delegate this part of the task to someone else in the family, take a book or a radio with you to the laundry room. Transfer the wet clothing to the dryers little by little, taking lots of rest breaks in between.

• **Dress for the workout that laundry is:** Laundry rooms in apartment buildings or house basements are often chilly. Make sure you are warm enough and comfortable. Wear clothing that is loose and layered. This helps you breathe and relax while you work.

• **Sorting:** This is often the toughest part of laundry for people with RSI. I know it was for me. If you have severe chronic pain, I suggest that you don't put your clothes away. Leave your laundry in the basket. If you are having company and don't want your clothes unfolded and out in the open, get someone to help!

• **Extra money:** If you live in the city, treat yourself to sending your laundry out to a service. Most will pick up, sort, and deliver. This is really worth it if you can afford it.

• **Remember to ask for help:** If you have a family, tell them they need to pitch in until you are better. Divide up the laundry tasks and delegate. It is in your family's best interest for you to recover as quickly as possible. A little extra effort on everyone's part will make everyone feel better. If you don't have family nearby, you can always ask a friend to help and have a productive visit.

Grocery Shopping

Many grocery stores even in the country will deliver food to your home if you explain that you are injured and can't carry packages. If not, I suggest you shop with a friend who can carry the packages. Strength building (lifting and carrying food bags) is one of the last levels of recovery you will achieve. It is a frustrating aspect of RSI—not being able to carry—but you can succeed in completing almost any carrying chore if you ask for help. Many stores today will have people walk down aisles with you and put things in your cart, put things on the check-out counter, and load your car if you need assistance. Ask the manager at the local grocery store if such help could be provided for you. You may be pleasantly surprised at the sensitive response.

Dishes and Cleanup

Here again, the whole trick is to look at what is causing you problems, replace any heavy dishes with lighter, more durable items, and then break down the task so it is RSI-friendly. Dish washing provides soothing warmth for your hands. Here are some suggestions on how you can make this task relaxing and enjoy the warm-water therapy it offers.

• **Find a comfortable height for your work.** If you find yourself lifting your arms or holding your arms up when doing the dishes, try standing on a step stool in front of your sink. The new angle it provides may be much more forgiving. Work with gravity as much as you can. In other words, don't lift when you can lower something down. Picking up something that is waist high is much easier than reaching up to a high counter and trying to take down a heavy dish.

• **Replace china or stoneware dishes, glasses, and silverware with plastics.** There are wonderful, attractive, *light* plastic dishes and silverware on the market that are a blessing to anyone with RSI. Besides being easy to handle, these plastic replacements will save your good dishes from falling victim to weak grips or uncontrollable motor coordination. With fancy napkins and a flower, you can make your table setting as attractive as it is healthy. In the catalogs listed in the appendices, you will find plastic bowls that also have rubber bottoms that grip the table so they don't move and are easier to use. Talk to your physical or occupational therapist about other tools that might help as you recover from RSI.

• **Buy a light skillet and saucepan.** With these two light pans, you can cook almost anything and go easy on your hands. Go to your local kitchen supply store and try out a couple. Ask for suggestions on light pans from the staff as there is usually a selection from which you can choose.

• **Soak dishes overnight.** Most RSI sufferers have more energy in the mornings. Tasks such as dish washing are best done at this high-energy point of the day.

• **Dish washing machines.** Here we have a double-edged sword: You don't have to scrub the dishes or hold them very long when you use a dishwasher, but the very act of putting the dishes in the machine is stressful and pulling them out after they are clean I found almost impossible. When my RSI was at its worst, I washed by hand whenever I could. If you want to use the machine, see if a step stool helps or try sitting in a chair as you remove the dishes. Try to move in big sweeping movements instead of tight, small ones. Another task-saving move is to leave the clean dishes in the machine and only take them out when you need them. To fight a large stack of dirty dishes in the sink, wash small batches in the machine. Last but not least, place ice and heat on your injuries after every dish washing. Throughout the task, remember to breathe deeply.

Making Your Bed

This daily task is incredibly strenuous work for anyone with RSI. First, consider how important it is to make your bed. If it is not really that important to you but just a habit, let it go. Just close the bedroom door and walk away. Use your energy on chores that are important to you. If you must make your bed to enjoy your day, make the bed while you are still in it. It is one way to get the job done with much less work. You can fluff the pillows into shape by gently kicking them. This is not only good exercise but it gets the job done effectively.

Putting on clean sheets or stripping a bed is another matter. If at all possible, have someone else do this for you while you are recovering from RSI. But if you must do it yourself, it is easier to strip a bed while you are still in it—rather than standing at the side, reaching, lifting, and pulling. When you remake the bed, do it in stages as you have learned to do everything else. Pacing is the key. Put one sheet on in the morning, and one on in the afternoon. You can put the blankets on when you climb into bed at night. Discuss how to put on pillowcases with your physical or occupational therapist.

Cleaning the Bathroom

Ah, it's great to take a nice hot bath in a sparkling-clean bathroom. But we all know how daunting a job it can be to keep it that way. Here is an easy way to keep your bathroom clean one little step at a time.

• Get in the tub to clean it rather than reaching over the side. Plan to get wet.

• Use big circles when you scrub the floor, the tub, or any surface. Stay away from those tiny, fine movements that greatly aggravate your RSI.

• Clean the sink one day, the floor the next, toilet the next, and shower/tub the last, then rotate back to the beginning so you will always have just one manageable chore to face and will always keep this room fresh.

• Always use a cleaner that requires no rinsing. This will cut your time and effort in half.

Getting Dressed

You need to experiment and decide which kind of fastening is easiest for you to use and incorporate that into your wardrobe for recovery. Buttons are often difficult and too numerous for most, but if you work in a corporate office, there may be a dress code requiring dress shirts. If you live with someone else, you can ask him to button your shirt almost completely and then slip it over your head. For other garments, try Velcro fasteners—often easier to manipulate for those with RSI. Others find zippers more friendly. And some adopt a clothing style with no fastening—shirts that slip over the head and pants with elastic waistbands. For any kind of clothing difficulty, look through the catalogs that can be ordered from the listings in the appendices. Also, ask your physical or occupational therapist for help. Shoelaces are often a big problem and actually have a simple solution. If you are wearing tie shoes, there are Spirolaces in white, black, blue, and pink. The laces are elastic spirals that, when laced on the shoe, require no tying and stay snug. Each pair, on sneakers, lasts for about nine to twelve months before becoming slightly slack. They only cost $3.95 a pair. Try them. If your experience is like mine, shoe tying is exhausting and difficult and these laces are a good energy-saving solution.

Now you have a good idea of how to approach tasks and break them down to be RSI friendly. But social situations can be just as difficult and a lot more embarrassing if you don't think them through ahead of time. The next chapter is all about how to cope and be comfortable with daily social situations when you have RSI.

12. RSI and Your Social Life

A simple handshake, a night at the movies, a romantic encounter with your lover, applauding at a Broadway show—all these everyday social actions can be pain inducing and embarrassing when you have RSI.

I hope what we share in this book will save you from discomfort by presenting solutions others have developed for these situations. The following suggestions came from occupational therapists and many RSI sufferers who offered them in the hope that you fare well and recover quickly.

The Handshake

Whether it's business or purely social, judgments about your character are often formed by the strength of your grip, the temperature and dryness of your hand, and the tension in your wrist when you shake hands with those you first meet. A lingering handshake can be the first step toward a romantic relationship or the end to the hope of one ever blossoming. Remember your girlfriends saying, "Oh, he's awful. I shook his hands and they were wet and clammy. And his wrist was all limp." If you don't shake hands, it is awkward at best and can be considered an insult or a rejection at worst. Offering one's open hand is a sign of willingness to begin, to meet on equal ground. Making an apology with no hand offered, despite the reason, often sets the stage for suspicion. Most of us with RSI don't wear splints, leaving our injuries invisible. Most of us look normal. Most people don't believe we can't use our hands and most aren't interested in our explanations.

Here are some solutions to overcome the handshake problem that have worked for others. Try several until you find one that fits your personal style.

• Wear a hand brace in social situations. People won't offer to shake your hand, and they won't be offended when you don't extend yours if your injury is visible.

• Adapt the European custom of kissing both cheeks in greeting.

• If you are with a close friend at a big event, put your arm around him when meeting people and tuck your other hand behind your back. Then nod and smile as you meet others.

• When someone offers his hand, place it horizontally between both of yours, like a sandwich, and gently squeeze his hand. This satisfies the other person, and suggests that you are sensitive, gentle, and straightforward. (You have symbolically enveloped their offering of friendship.) Make sure you look the person straight in the eyes as you do this.

• Women: You can, in certain informal and friendly circumstances, offer your hand to be kissed, not shaken, with a half smile.

• Men: You, too, can take on the role of Hollywood gallant by kissing or air kissing the back of a woman's hand.

Applauding and Other Audience Behaviors

Applauding is painful when you have RSI. The purpose of applauding is to show appreciation to the performers, but it is also a way to share your enjoyment with the rest of the audience. Try faking it and applaud without touching your hands. Usually, there is so much sound around you, people will assume you are clapping as loud as they are. They don't care how much noise you make. In operas and classical concerts, stamping your feet is an acceptable way to show your appreciation. For pop concerts, giving a holler usually suffices.

Movies and Concerts

Public seating is notoriously uncomfortable for those with RSI. Here are some suggestions on how to make yourself more comfortable physically and socially.

- **Bring pillows.** Don't be shy. Bring enough to be comfortable.
- **Sit on the aisle.** This allows you to shift your position often to keep your hands, arms, neck, and shoulders relaxed and comfortable without jarring those around you.
- **Open your option to stand up.** Explain to your seat partner that you may get up and stand in the back of the auditorium during the concert for a while. Standing room is great for those with RSI. You can slip out the door and stretch when necessary and the narrow seats no longer will push you into a painful position.
- **Wear comfortable, warm clothing and bring a scarf.** Air-conditioning often creates drafts on the neck and shoulders that will incite muscle contractions. Know where your cold spots are and, if one of them is your hands, bring gloves if necessary. Wear comfortable, supportive shoes. If you wind up standing a lot in the back, your whole body will appreciate it.
- **Use intermission to stretch.** Find a hallway to do your stretches during intermission. I was pleasantly surprised recently at a concert when I made my way into a hallway to stretch and found two men in tails doing stretches as well.

Holding Hands

Place your hand on top of your partner's. Then he or she doesn't have to remember not to squeeze and you still have physical contact. Explain to your partner that entwining fingers is painful. Try to express yourself clearly so he or she will sense your affection without misinterpreting your gestures as rejections. Even if you are not used to verbalizing these things, start doing it. Your relationship will become stronger as you both understand more about each other's needs and desires.

Transportation

As a passenger with RSI, you may experience pain and discomfort simply from the vibration of moving vehicles in which you travel. Bring pillows to buffer and dull them. Also, take periodic stops during a long trip. Get out and walk around at least every half hour. This should help cut down on muscle spasms and cramps to which you may be prone. Your regular movements will keep the blood flowing and keep that oxygen pulsing through your system.

Sit on the aisle in trains and buses. This way you can walk around or stand up and stretch periodically. Try to avoid seats right over the motor as the vibrations will be worse there. In a bus, this usually means you should avoid the backseat.

As a driver, you will need more frequent breaks than the passengers. Holding a steering wheel is a static, fine-motor activity full of direct and aggravating vibrations. The handlebars of a bicycle or motorcycle are worse as your body's forced into even more awkward, unnatural static postures. Gel-lined gloves found in some of the catalogs in the back of this book will help reduce the discomfort of these vibrations. Wheelchair users who have similar hand problems due to overuse injuries have worn these gloves for years.

If your RSI is quite pronounced, you may find long trips extremely stressful until you really begin to recover. If you must take a trip, try to limit them to day trips that involve lots of walking or short social events where you can sit and stand as needed.

Parties and Invitations

Watch out for standing around at cocktail parties with a drink in one hand and food in the other. This is a very stressful position. Stand near a table where you can rest your glass and plate. Walk around. Come back to it. Keep changing positions.

Your social life will not cease just because you are injured. Again, clear communication is the key to keeping friends and avoiding misunderstandings that just increase the stress in your life. If you decline an invitation, make sure that you explain that you are not up to it but would love to see them another time. If you want to give a dinner party, make it a potluck party. Or better yet, if you can afford it, take friends out to dinner. The more control you have over your environment during the painful stages of RSI, the more comfortable you will be. If you are at a friend's house or a party, don't be shy about borrowing a sweater from your host if you are cold. Go home early with a clear "Lovely time. Glad I could make it. I need to rest now." You don't need everyone to understand all the complexities of your limitations. You just need them to understand you enjoyed your time with them but have special needs now.

Isolation

RSI breeds fatigue, pain, and depression as you know. You may feel as if you don't want to socialize at all. Make the effort to stay in contact with friends and family. Isolating yourself can only deepen your depression and pain. Socializing is a form of distraction. You need to feel your loved ones care about you during this difficult time. If you can't handle big gatherings, go out for tea with a friend. Find a walking partner. Expressing interest in a friend's life is the best way to build the friendship and find the emotional support you seek. The love and support offered by family and friends will help you heal and feel better about yourself. Open up to them, don't shut them out.

RSI and Intimacy

Communication, creativity, patience, and honesty are the successful keys to any intimate relationship. When you are injured, they are even more important. If you've never talked about your feelings and preferences before, it's time to learn. If you find this awkward or difficult, make it a game with your partner. You can each start with a simple statement and gradually add vocabulary that will help you express your needs and desires verbally for all your intimate situations. A typical RSI intimate encounter often sounds like this for the uninitiated: The RSI sufferer mutters, "Mmmm. Yes. Ouch!" The uninjured, aroused partner may respond, "Yes. Right. What? I hurt you? Oh, God, I didn't mean to hurt you! I thought . . ." Naturally, this can break a romantic mood and make it seem impossible to rekindle. Couples often get to the point where there is so much anger, rejection, and confusion that the relationship falls apart. The way to prevent this is to talk.

The challenge is to open up, face the challenges of RSI together, and discover the solutions to the problems *together*. If you find the couch more comfortable than your shared bed, buy a bigger bed or explain the reason you are moving to the couch to your partner. Express yourself so that your partner doesn't feel so lonely and isolated. Instead of "Ouch!" try "Yes, that's good, but I just need to adjust a little. There, that's better." This lets your partner know that this position causes discomfort and the other is comfortable. Experiment. Try everything from adding pillows for support to using humor when you move into an intimate space with one another. Talk about everything openly and honestly. Most of all, remember to be respectful of each other's feelings.

Many partners need the illusion of *spontaneity* to instigate an intimate encounter. When you have RSI, spontaneity is often not possible. However, there are steps you can take that will help you get into a warm, loving mood and ease your pain as well. You can take a warm bath, do gentle stretching, and think to save your energy during the day when you expect a sexual encounter that evening. These all will help you optimize your energy and ability to move without pain. You don't always have to tell the other person about your preparation. That is the illusion. Or make the warming up part of foreplay. Two can take a bath or shower and warm up. Your uninjured partner can help you limber and stretch and relax both of you by talking and teasing. You can also take a shower together afterward. Let your partner wash your hair and massage your tired shoulders and arms. Just remember that a little love and creativity can go a long way.

There is also frustration because some partners feel "neglected." Many times one partner of a married couple will complain: "I have to do all the work!" This makes everyone feel guilty and resentful and angry. Even with RSI, you can hug your partner or respond verbally. You have a mouth and legs that can stroke and kiss. Explore. Create. Talk. Don't let comments like the one above slide away without resolution. If you need help communicating, go to a counselor who will help you clear up any misunderstandings and find other ways to resolve conflicts.

Understanding Responsibility

As a polio and RSI survivor, I finally learned that it is *my* responsibility to express myself when I am in pain. Voicing discomfort is different from complaining. Sometimes my partner would misunderstand my change in mood or sudden sharpness in tone as an out-of-the-blue form of irritability. And, logically, he thought the change was because of him. When I learned to tell my partner my neck was starting to burn and the pain was making me a little tired or that, suddenly, my fingers were numb or there was tingling starting up and down my arm, our relationship began to improve. He made suggestions on how to accommodate my discomfort and still share in an activity. I began to recognize what made me tired and triggered pain and what didn't. I began to recover by retraining myself with the help of my partner. He felt good because he was taking care of me by finding things he could do to help me feel better. I felt independent and good because I had expressed my needs and was cared for. We both felt better because we had communicated our feelings and helped each other understand.

Don't get me wrong. This is not always easy going. However, communicating clearly with your partner will help you recover if you work at it. At best, you'll have a loving ally during your recuperation. You also have to learn that while your partner doesn't need to hear you complain all the time, he or she does need to know how you feel. You are human and are allowed to complain, but put yourself in your partner's place. You also need to express interest in his or her well-being and what is happening to him or her. You need to care for your partner. You may feel lousy but asking about how your partner feels may make you feel better.

It will distract from your pain. Remember to focus on your partner's needs regularly for both your sakes.

The Unbelieving Partner

I was blessed with a husband who emotionally and intellectually believed in my injury and in my degree of pain. Many people aren't as lucky and have spouses or partners who doubt the severity and pain of RSI. There are counselors and support groups for partners of RSI sufferers. I suggest before you go running to outside help, try using analogies with which your partner can identify such as "Imagine how you would feel if someone was stabbing invisible needles into your arms and neck and instead of sympathizing, I just got annoyed. Imagine if I didn't believe you? How would you feel?" Another analogy that may bring your experience home to your partner is referring to a past injury of his or hers. For example, "Remember last year when you sprained your wrist badly but still went to your computer job? Remember how painful it was every time you tried to use your hand? But only you could feel the pain. No one else could see your injury. Imagine how you would feel if I ignored your pain or didn't believe you and said, 'You've got to be kidding? I've worked all day and now you want me to hang pictures? You take care of it!'" While you're apart, think up analogies like these to clarify specific instances when your partner misunderstood.

One woman told me that she didn't want to be put in the position of *counseling* her husband. She was a social worker and she didn't want to work at home. She expected her husband to understand without any explanation. Well, let's face it. We all counsel each other. And relationships are work. If we want them to stay strong and grow, we need continually to teach each other about ourselves.

The Power of Humor

Communication doesn't necessarily have to be confrontational. One of the strongest rescuing factors that helped my husband and me through the chronic years of my RSI was humor. Our ability to see the lighter side of a crisis saved our marriage. When things got really tough, we sat back and talked about all the good parts of each other. We were lucky enough to be able to laugh about our mistakes. And when a situation or issue seemed complicated and insurmountable, we sat back and reminded each other about what was important. We had a comfortable apartment and he worked at a job he enjoyed. I was retraining my muscles and learning how to move with less pain. And, most important, we had each other. During a long recovery that is typical of many RSI sufferers, a positive attitude can save the day.

Recognize that your injury creates stress for both of you. Find activities that offer enjoyment and comfort for both of you. Realize that you each need a vacation from the rigors of RSI. Take breaks from the intensity of your injury and talk of other things besides the therapy, support groups, or political actions you may be involved in. Talk about vacation plans, your family, and other important aspects of life. Don't let RSI monopolize all your energy and time.

Birth-Control Methods

When your hands don't work, birth-control devices can be cumbersome and often impossible to manipulate. Below are some extra information and tips about the various methods on the market for those women with RSI.

The Birth-Control Pill

The pill is a physician-prescribed drug that prevents unwanted pregnancies with one pill a day. However, it can also cause water retention and swelling of the connective tissues, which results in pain for those with RSI. If you want to use the pill, ask your gynecologist to closely monitor you. If discomfort occurs, discuss other options with your doctor.

Mechanical Methods

These include the diaphragm, the IUD (intrauterine device), and condoms. They are often difficult to use because they require fine-motor control and strength in the fingers, hands, and wrists—all the areas affected by RSI.

• *The diaphragm:* The best method for introducing and extracting a diaphragm is having your partner help. You can make the insertion of the diaphragm an integral and enjoyable part of foreplay. The more you relax, the easier it is to introduce the device into the body. The manufacturers recently took the *diaphragm introducer* off the market because not enough women were buying it. However, speak to your physician; he or she may have some samples stockpiled in his office. The introducer takes the stress off the hands and, if you have weakened muscles, will do most of the work for you. A woman with RSI shares her experience:

> When I first got RSI, my fingers and hands were so weak I could barely unbutton my blouse, let alone take out or put in my diaphragm. But it wasn't something I thought about until I tried to remove it and couldn't. I wound up going to my gynecologist and having her remove it. That cost me seventy-five bucks! Then I talked to my occupational therapist and she suggested I ask my partner for help. I can tell you, I've never had to pay another seventy-five dollars and my sex life improved!

To remove your diaphragm: Take a warm bath. The warmth helps relax your muscles so you can pull the diaphragm out easier. During the acute stage and with particular kinds of RSI, this may still be impossible for a while. Communicate with your partner. Ask for help. If you really get stuck, you can, for a fee, like the woman above, go to a clinic where a doctor will remove it for you. Extracting the diaphragm after six to eight hours is important so that an infection or irritation doesn't develop.

• *The IUD:* Depending on your age and reproductive wishes for the future, the IUD (intrauterine device) may be suitable. It releases no chemicals and is inserted by your physician. There is no need to remove it; however, it should be checked yearly. Some women have increased yeast infections with the IUD just because there is a foreign body lodged in their system. Make sure you speak to the doctor about its potential drawbacks.

• *The condom:* There is always the condom, which the male partner can slip on himself. This method, although easy for women with RSI, is not as effective in preventing pregnancy as other methods if used alone.

Chemical Methods

These are somewhat problematic because they involve the release of excess progesterone. *Depo-Provera*, which is injected every three months, and the *Norplant patch* fall into this category. As mentioned before, progesterone has many side effects that may negatively impact RSI.

Conclusion

The ball is now in your court. You've educated yourself and have the means to recover. You've learned how to relax those painful muscle spasms and stretch your contracted tendons. When you're tired and in pain, you know how to reduce the inflammation with ice packs and increase your circulation through limbering and yoga. You have begun to explore all the possible therapies available and are exercising each morning and evening before bed. You are putting aside time every day to walk and revitalize your whole system. You've adjusted your diet so your body is finally getting the nutrients it needs to heal. You've defined your comfort zone and know how to pace yourself at work and at home.

You should begin to feel better just because you are taking such an active role in your fight to overcome RSI. You are beginning to express your needs and find support and are developing a new and healthier lifestyle. As you use our eight-step healing program over the next year, we hope you continue to learn and grow. We feel privileged to have shared our expertise and experiences with you. May you soon be healthy and back to work.

Reading List

1. Anderson, Bob. *Stretching at Your Computer or Desk*. Shelter Publications, Inc., 1997.
2. Baldwin, Fred, and Suzanne McInerney. *Infomedicine: A Consumer's Guide to the Latest Medical Research*. Little, Brown, and Company, 1996.
3. Benson, Herbert, M.D., with Marg Stark. *Timeless Healing: The Power and Biology of Belief*. Simon and Schuster/Fireside Book, 1996.
4. Bucci, Luke, Ph.D. *Pain Free: The Definitive Guide to Healing Arthritis, Low-Back Pain, and Sports Injuries through Nutrition and Supplements*. The Summit Group, 1995.
5. Lasater, Judith, Ph.D., PT. *Relax and Renew: Restful Yoga for Stressful Times*. Rodmell Press, 1995.
6. McIlwain, Harris H., M.D., and Debra Fulghum Bruce. *The Fibromyalgia Handbook*. Owl Books/Henry Holt and Company, 1996.
7. Morgan, Brian L. G., M.D. *Nutrition Prescription: Strategies for Preventing and Treating 50 Common Diseases*. Gallagher/Howard Associates and Royal Tree Enterprises, Inc., 1987.
8. Morton, Mary, and Michael Morton. *Five Steps to Selecting the Best Alternative Medicine: A Guide to Complementary and Integrative Health Care*. New World Library, 1996.
9. Peddie, Sandra, and Craig H. Rosenberg, M.D. *The Repetitive Strain Injury Sourcebook*. Lowell House, 1997.
10. Siegel, Bernie, M.D. *How to Live Between Office Visits*. Harper and Row Publishers, 1993.
11. ———. *Love, Medicine and Miracles*. Harper and Row Publishers, 1986.

Internet Resources

The following resources include databases and electronic information sources to help you keep up with new developments, research, and support groups related to repetitive strain injuries.

Traditional Medical Resources

The **U.S. National Library of Medicine (NLM)** offers a few sites to help you stay current on the medical world's research findings on RSI. The home page is *http://www.nlm.nih.gov*. From there you can jump to any of the following:

- **HSTAT** is an invaluable site providing the full text of selected documents, including clinical practice guidelines, technology assessments, consensus conference reports, and treatment protocols.
- **Medline*plus*** is their new (Fall '98) easy-to-understand resource for the public. There are links here to self-help groups, access to National Institute of Health consumer-related organizations, clearinghouses, health-related organizations, and clinical trials. The site is continually updated and enhanced. The pages provide selected lists of resources, not a comprehensive listing. This is a free service.
- **PubMed** is a free World Wide Web (www) server for searching MEDLINE, also from NLM. **TOXNET** is also on the Web providing free toxicological information.

If you are looking for an address on the Internet, begin with *www.WHOIS*—an Internet address searcher. Medical resources on the Web are multiplying with amazing rapidity. Almost any issue of *Medical Matrix News*, an on-line newsletter, will list dozens of new medical resources you might want to explore.

The **American Academy of Neurology** publishes an on-line newsletter, *NeuroVista*, covering neurology, health, and wellness information. To access this newsletter go to *www.aan.com*.

The **Food and Drug Administration**'s home page is *http://www.fda.gov* and it offers links to other sources for government and nongovernmental resources concerning food and nutritional, chemical, biological, and technical information. To report serious adverse effects and product problems to MEDWATCH (a branch of the FDA) call 1-800-FDA-1088.

The **Health Care Financing Administration** (HCFA) created a Web site at *http://www.medicare.gov*. The departments include Medicare, managed care, who to contact, publications, wellness, fraud, and abuse. Those of you applying for social security disability will want to educate yourself using this site.

Through the **Johns Hopkins Health Information Center** on the Web you can receive a daily newsletter by subscribing to Intelihealth Newsletter at *http://www.intelihealth.com/signup?r+EMIHCOOO* or *http://www.intelihealth.com/signup?r=EMIHCOOO</A>*. Besides gathering the latest breaking scientific news from all over the world, the Johns Hopkins site also provides articles on different specific conditions and diseases. For general comments and questions E-mail them at *comments@intelihealth.com*.

The **U.S. Department of Health and Human Services** publishes an Internet newsletter covering the most recent proposals, laws passed, and discussions regarding food, drugs, and nutritional supplements. To reach it, go to **HHNEWS** at *http://www.fda.gov.bbs/topics/NEWS/NEW00637.html*.

Alternative Medicine Resources

General Alternative Medicine: *http:/www.Halcyon.com/Libastyr/netbib.html* and/or *http://www-hsl.mcmaster.ca/tomflem/altmed.html*.
Health World Online: *http://www.healthy.net*.
Holistic Internet Resources: *http://hir.com*.

Medication on-line information: *http://pharminfo.com* or *http://www.mcc.ac.uk./ pharmweb* or *http://www.wilmington.net/dees.*

Nutritional/diet information: *http://www.naludsa.gov.fnic.html* or *http://www. usda.gov* or *http://www.lifelines.com/ntnlnk.html* or *http://www.eatright.org.*

Yahoo Health: Alternative Medicine: *http://www.yahoo.com/Health/Alternative_ Medicine/.*

General Information Internet Sites

Repetitive strain injuries are also classified as cumulative trauma disorders (CTD) and musculoskeletal disease so also search under these umbrellas. Here is a list of noncommercial Internet resources that provide plain and simple information about RSI/CTDs:

Agency for Health Care Policy and Research (AHCPR): *http://www.ahcpr.gov/ news/press/lowback.htm.*

FAQ Typing Injury: *http://www.tifaq.com.*

Florida State University: *http://www.cs.fsu.edu.carpal.html.*

National Institute of Arthritis and Musculoskeletal and Skin Diseases: *http:// www.nih.gov/niams/healthinfo/.*

New York Academy of Medicine: *http://www.nyam.org/library/medcenter.html/.* On-line access to one of the largest medical libraries in the United States, with a collection that includes nearly 705,000 volumes, 275,000 portraits and illustrations, and 182,000 pamphlets.

RSI-UK: *http://www.demon.co.uk/rsi/.*

RXList: *http://www.rxlist.com/.* In-depth profiles of 500 prescription drugs including approximately 90 percent of what is on the market and under development in the United States. This is presently the on-line medical community's drug reference source.

University of Nebraska: *http://engr-www.unl.edu/ee/eeshop/rsi.html .*

Your Legal Rights

For more information concerning your legal rights and the Americans with Disabilities Act (ADA) contact *http://www.public.iastate.edu/~sbilling/ada.html/.* Telephone number for ADA information: 1-800-ADA-9675.

E-mail Lists

RSI-UK is a more broad-based discussion group. Send a message containing the text *join-rsi-uk* to this address, *RSI-UK-ADMIN@loud-n-clear.com .*

    Sorehand is a discussion group primarily about carpal tunnel syndrome and tendinitis. To join, send a message with the text *SIGNON SOREHAND firstname surname* to *LISTSERV@ITSSRV1.UCSF.EDU. .*

Organizations,
Government Agencies,
Libraries, and Newsletters

Organizations and Government Agencies

American Occupational Therapy Association: 301-948-9626. This association refers employers and individuals with disabilities to occupational therapists for help with job performance analysis, identifying job accommodations and modifications. They also have local chapters throughout the United States.

Association of Occupational and Environmental Clinics (AOEC): 202-347-4676. AOEC can refer you to the nearest clinic that will treat your work-related health problem. They are open Monday through Friday, nine to five, eastern standard time.

Equal Employment Opportunity Commission (EEOC): 1-800-669-4000. This office will discuss and help you file a complaint concerning workplace health problems or any kind of discrimination or harassment including denial by employers of high-risk ergonomic situations. They are open twenty-four hours a day.

Job Accommodation Network (JAN): 1-800-526-7234 or 1-800-ADA-WORK. This network provides free consulting by professional human factors/ergonomic counselors about work-site accommodations.

National Foundation for Osteoporosis: 1-800-464-6700. For those of you with both RSI and osteoporosis, this source may be invaluable. Their headquarters is in the Washington, D.C., area.

National Institute for Occupational Safety and Health (NIOSH): 1-800-669-4000. NIOSH was set up to research occupational safety and health. If you have an unusual problem that the state office (OSHA) cannot address, call the national institute. They have the power to inspect the work site and make recommendations. They have *no enforcement powers*. They can, however, provide information on a variety of subjects, including national laws, and they have a continuing educational program.

National Women's Health Resource Center: 202-293-6045. This is a general clearinghouse for national resources specifically concerning women.

Occupational Safety and Health Administration (OSHA): This is the state office responsible for occupational safety and health. They can *inspect and enforce* workplace safety regulations. They also offer *free consultations* to small businesses. Office hours are Monday through Friday, from nine to five, eastern standard time. Your local office is in your phone book under *U.S. Government Offices: Occupational Safety and Health*.

Office of Occupational Medicine: 202-219-5003. This is an OSHA-consulting firm for physicians who want more detailed information about an occupational illness or injury. You may want to tell your doctor about this source if he or she has any questions. Their hours are Monday through Friday, eight to five, eastern standard time.

Research Institute for Human Engineering (Forschungsinstitut für Anthropotechnik-FAT): Telephone number: (+49) 228 94 35 10; fax number: (+49) 228 94 35 508; E-mail address: doering@fgan.de. This is a German institute with a staff of more than fifty employees. Most of the staff is fluent in both German and English. They study the relationship between, and adaptations necessary for, humans and machine systems. They develop ergonomic designs of complex human-machine systems including personnel ergonomics, which deal with personnel selection and training. Their programs also focus on environmental ergonomics, which deal with environmental factors that impact the workplace such as climate, light, and noise. Their workplace design department and man-machine dialogue department (MMD) can be quite helpful to small businesses in the United States that are searching for the most recent series of studies about environments that prevent RSI.

The RSI/Carpal Tunnel Syndrome Association: You can contact them at P.O. Box 514, Santa Rosa, CA 95402. This association is a clearinghouse for information about RSI. They publish a newsletter and keep a list of RSI support groups around the country.

Your union: Your union may be a good starting point if you are injured or feel your job site creates a high health risk. Ask to speak to the health and safety officer. He or she may know of other local, national, and international resources you may need to contact.

Massage and Body Work Resources

The Alexander Technique: 212-799-0468 (The New York Center) or 212-866-5640 (The North American Society of Teachers of the Alexander Technique) or write to The Society of Teachers of the Alexander Technique, 10 London House, 266 Fulham Road, London SW109EL, England.

The American Association of Acupuncture and Oriental Medicine: 919-787-5181 or write to 4101 Lake Bone Trail #201, Raleigh, North Carolina 27607-6518.

American Massage Therapy Association (AMTA): 708-864-0123.

The Feldenkrais Guild: 1-800-755-2118 or 514-926-0981.

The National Commission for the Certification of Acupuncturists: You can write them c/o National Acupuncture Headquarters, 1424 16th Street, N.W., Suite 501, Washington, DC 10036.

Libraries

There is a national network of medical libraries that you can use. If you want to learn about a particular medical condition or procedure, these regional offices will direct you to the most appropriate medical library in your area. Find which region includes your state and call. Many also have on-line access so ask for that address when you contact them.

Region 1: DE, NJ, NY, PA: 212-876-8763.

Region 2: AL, DC, FL, GA, MD, MS, NC, SC, TN, VA, WV, the Virgin Islands, and Puerto Rico: 401-328-2855.

Region 3: IA, IL, IN, KY, MI, MN, ND, OH, SD, WI: 312-996-2464.
Region 4: CO, KS, MO, NE, UT, WY: 402-559-4326.
Region 5: AR, LA, NM, OK, TX: 713-790-7053.
Region 6: AK, ID, MT, OR, WA: 206-543-8262.
Region 7: AZ, CA, HI, NV, and Territories of the Pacific Basin: 301-825-1200.
Region 8: CT, MA, ME, NH, RI, VT: 203-679-4500.

Newsletters

CTD News: 1-800-554-4283. This is an industry-oriented newsletter published ten times a year that covers cumulative trauma disorders including those from noncomputer sources. It is a particularly good source for legal, insurance, and regulatory information. You can write them at 10 Railroad Avenue, P.O. Box 239, Haverford, PA 19041-0239. The subscription cost is $125.00.

The Healthy Office Report targets information about workplace health issues for clerical professions. It covers RSI, sick building syndrome, and sexual harassment. The cost is $35.00 for twelve issues. You can write them at 54 West Hubbard Street, Suite 403, Chicago, IL 60610.

Repetitive Stress Injury Litigation Reporter: 1-800-345-1101. This newsletter covers court rulings on RSI lawsuits all over the United States. Court documents are available upon request. The cost is $550.00 a year for twelve issues, $325.00 for six issues/six months. You can also write them at 1646 West Chester Pike, P.O. Box 1000, Westtown, PA 19395.

Workplace Safety and Health: This newsletter reports on federal initiatives, OSHA proclamations, national legislation, and corporate practices relating to workplace health and safety. The subscription cost is $35.00 a year for twelve issues. You can reach them at Courthouse Place, 54 West Hubbard Street, Suite 403, Chicago, IL 60610.

Note: There are many other newsletters concerning RSI health, alternative medicine treatments, and other issues on the Internet. See the Internet Resources Appendix.

Catalogs

The following companies offer products and exercise equipment used in daily living (kitchen, bathroom, and bed accessories, exercise balls, wrist braces, etc.):

Sammons "Enrichments": 1-800-323-5547.
AliMed: 1-800-225-2610.
North Coast: 1-800-821-9319.
Maxi Aids and Appliances for Independent Living (computers, accessories, clocks, etc.): 1-800-522-6294.

To find a product or manufacturer: There is a wonderful database called **Abledata** (NARRIC). It is updated daily. Contact them (phone number: 1-800-227-0216; fax number: 1-301-587-1967) with an idea of the product you need or the manufacturer you're looking for and they will do a search for you while you wait.

Before you buy anything to help ease your daily routine from these catalogs, *check with your occupational or physical therapist.* He or she often has demos for you to try before you buy a product. Talk to him or her and discuss your needs and get feedback on brands, sizes, weight restrictions, and other product specifications. Then, call the catalog from which you wish to order and, before you make your purchase, talk to the customer service representative regarding:

• *Return policies:* Make sure you understand the length of time you have if you want to return. Find out what the company policy is regarding refunds: Will they give you a full refund, store credit, or partial credit? Are you responsible for handling and processing charges on the other end? Under what conditions will they accept a return?

• *Product specifications:* Even if you don't see what you need in the catalog, ask if they carry what you want. Ask for specific dimensions, color, price, and weight. Ask the customer service representative's opinion about the product: Have they had good feedback about the product? Is it returned a lot?

• *Warranty policies:* Some products have a six-month or one-year warranty attached to the product. Some have none at all. If the product is a machine or has many parts, ask if there is a service center near you or whether you will have to pack it up and send it back for repairs.

Index